Understanding the Horse's Back

UNDERSTANDING
The Horse's Back

Sara Wyche

CROWOOD

First published in 1998 by
The Crowood Press Ltd
Ramsbury, Marlborough
Wiltshire SN8 2HR

British Library Cataloguing-in-Publication Data

A catalogue record for this book is available from the British Library.

ISBN 1 86126 114 4

Dedication
To Jim.

Credits
Photographs and line-drawings by the author.

Typeset and designed by Phoenix Typesetting, Ilkley, West Yorkshire.

Printed and bound in Great Britain by Redwood Books, Trowbridge, Wiltshire

Contents

Acknowledgements

In a small town in Germany lives a man who breeds horses. Nothing remarkable in that. He also breaks them in and competes on them. Nothing remarkable in that either. Like all breeders and riders his horses have their fair share of problems. What makes this person special is that *his* horses never have back problems! Not through luck, lack of judgement, and certainly not through ignorance; this is simply a horseman who has an overwhelming sense of responsibility towards the movements of the horse – to preserve their natural rhythm and flow, whatever the level of training and whatever the type of work. There are no concessions to rider error, no concessions to the degree of collection. Short, fumbling strides are not only unacceptable, they are inexcusable. The horse must carry its rider willingly forwards, with a back that is soft and supple, and limbs that swing freely and comfortably. Whether it takes twenty minutes or two hours, the horse does not return to the stable until its back moves with *Schwung*.

It has taken me a whole veterinary degree and twelve years of treating horses with back disorders, to appreciate fully the importance of *Schwung*. It is the most fundamental characteristic of the horse's natural movements, and the quality most easily lost as soon as the horse has to carry a rider. This book has come into being because one man in Germany insisted that his horses' backs never lost their swing!

Introduction ———————————————

'If you prick us, do we not bleed? If you tickle us, do we not laugh? . . . And if you wrong us, shall we not revenge?'

William Shakespeare: *The Merchant of Venice*

In the thirteenth century, Mongolian warriors rode thousands of miles across Asia on horseback. To tenderize their meat, they used to put large slabs of it under their saddles. Did their horses all end up with back problems? The answer is, probably not as many as those horses of ours that work for only a few hours a week, but in enclosed spaces and on entirely unsuitable surfaces, or else spend a great deal of time standing on one spot in the confines of a stable. It's all a question of balance: physical balance, mental balance, emotional balance and, who knows, probably spiritual balance as well.

In human medicine, back pain is often regarded as something of an enigma. There are sources of back pain – such as slipped discs, fractures, compression of the spinal cord, or arthritis – which can be demonstrated by modern imaging techniques, but what about those subtle variations in muscle tone, or slight deviations in posture? Small areas of muscle tension cannot be made visible by X-rays, yet they may significantly interrupt the flow of information between a muscle and its nerve, and thus restrict the freedom of movement throughout the whole body.

The presence of back pain in horses is disputed, both among riders and veterinarians. It shouldn't be. Pain is a nerve signal which is transmitted when specific chemicals are released in tissue that is threatened or damaged. This can happen in a back, just as it happens in a leg or a foot. However, when the painful site is in the horse's back, close to the spinal cord which is a direct link to the brain, and yet the horse is conditioned to show basic obedience to the rider, the behavioural expression of that pain can be extremely varied. Acute pain can lead to the most exaggerated response, like bolting or rearing; chronic pain can be suppressed to the extent that it is hard to demonstrate the existence of a problem at all. In horses, the enigma is not so much in the pain but in its cause. What was the situation that led to the misunderstanding, that caused the imbalance, that resulted in the damage, that triggered the signal? At what point did the problem become the pain?

Back pain is not new. Treatment of human back pain has preoccupied civilizations for centuries. At present, in the twentieth century, our treatment is largely based on chemical pain control or surgery, yet previous civilizations developed entire philosophies of life to explain the phenomenon of pain in the human

7

back. These philosophies went far beyond any simple medical definition. The great, ancient civilizations of the world all regarded the back as an interface between the living energy of the human being and the energy of the world around him. The back's physical health depended on the human's mental, emotional and spiritual state. If there was no pain, the body must be in harmony with its surroundings; if there was pain, the body must be at odds, either with its emotions, or with its life-style.

Today, more working hours are lost to industry through back pain than through any other cause. Although we are beginning to realize the importance of postural comfort, both at home, in the car, and in the workplace, our high-speed, high-tech life-style doesn't always allow sufficient time for us to put this knowledge into practice. Not so very long ago, one way to close the door on the pressures of a hectic environment was to enter into the company of a horse, to experience the world from the vantage point of an animal with a single-horse-power engine and a top speed of 30 m.p.h. Now it seems we have drawn the horse into our own world: instead of leaving behind our own busy schedules, we simply add our horses to the agenda, fitting them into an already overflowing timetable.

It is therefore almost inevitable that the horse's back should come under the influence of the same problems that affect his human partner. The whole anatomy of the human spine acts directly upon that of the horse. It transmits the commands for equestrianism, but it cannot help transmitting a whole range of human emotions at the same time. We all know that a rider's anxiety will be felt through the saddle, and that a 'plod' may wake up under an 'electric backside', but the spectrum of human emotion is much wider than this, and the horse is a very sensitive recipient.

Diagnosing back problems in horses is not without its difficulties because so many factors have to be taken into consideration. For example, humans are free to take off any shoes or clothing that make them feel uncomfortable. The horse can only try to communicate his discomfort by changing the way he moves, or by making small changes to his facial expression. If early signs of discomfort are overlooked the symptoms can accumulate until the back is thrown out of balance. The result is a back problem, even though the source is not necessarily in the back.

Producing hard, visual evidence for every case of suspected back pain in horses is usually beyond the scope of general veterinary practice, and often beyond the financial scope of many horse owners. The sophisticated diagnostic procedures used in human medicine are available for horses, but because of the size of the patient and the cost of the equipment, they are only to be found at specialist equine clinics. Enter the back person. Once upon a time this was someone who manually adjusted elements of the horse's spine using a basic knowledge of levers. Nowadays, a back person may be any one of a number of therapists who not only manipulate without apparent physical force but who talk of harmonizing energy and expanding auras!

Orthodox medicine addresses the problems in backs by using chemical or surgical pain relief. However, there is currently a growing concern about the role of posture and emotion in the development of back pain. Ancient forms of medicine are increasingly sought after because they take into consideration the effect of the patient's emotional state on his otherwise physical illness. This holistic approach to treatment is the basis for acupuncture and acupressure, as well as the more recently derived therapies such as homoeopathy, chiropractic and osteopathy. These alternative forms of medicine are now being successfully used to help horses with a variety of locomotor problems. In fact, there is almost an excess of alternative therapies available for horses, which has led to something of a therapeutic free-for-all. Whilst many disorders in the back certainly benefit from treatment with non-orthodox medicine, there is unfortunately a tendency to circumvent an exact diagnosis – sometimes at the expense of the horse.

It is often said that the horse's back was never designed to carry a rider. This is rather like saying that if God had meant man to fly, He would have given him wings. The horse's back is a complex web of muscles and ligaments around a hollow, bony core, which protects the nerves vital to every function in the body. The horse is a natural athlete, and there is no reason why he should not continue to be an athlete in partnership with a human being, provided he is skilfully and considerately trained. All we have to remember is that beneath the saddle there is living tissue, *not* a collection of mechanical bits and pieces.

1 What is a Back? ───

What is the difference between a crocodile, a jellyfish, and a salmon? Did an antelope ever need an osteopath, or a camel a chiropractor? They all have backs of some description, backs that are highly mobile and that perform great feats of strength and agility. Why is it unlikely that these backs will ever need the same sort of attention paid to the back of the human – or the back of the horse? What exactly is a back, and what makes the horse's and the human's back special?

The major division in the animal kingdom is made between those creatures that have backbones and those that do not: the vertebrates and invertebrates. Vertebrae developed for two reasons: first, to provide a stable, central axis for the whole musculoskeletal system and, second, to protect the nerve-fibres needed to operate not only this system, but all the internal organs. When life crawled out of the primeval swamp, it needed an efficient means of getting about on dry land. This led to a gradual lengthening of the limbs, as well as changes in neck length, skull weight, and tail strength. It all depended on what height your dinner was from the ground, and how fast and manoeuvrable you needed to be to catch it. The more complex the range of movements, the more refined and highly tuned the musculoskeletal system became. We have only to think of the speed and

agility of the cheetah, or watch the domestic cat walk along a wall half the width of its own body, to appreciate that the specifications for these types of locomotor system – including the forces acting on the backbone – are going to be very different to those needed by a rhinoceros or a high-yield milk cow.

The evolutionary process has led to the creation of some bizarre and, at the same time, marvellous animal shapes. Yet evolution has always maintained a strict correlation between the shape of the body and its stability. If you have a heavy head and a cumbersome body, you will also have short sturdy legs, splayed feet, or some other form of counterweight, such as a powerful tail. If you are going to take your body swinging through the trees at high altitude, a prehensile tail becomes an extra limb for security. If you have a long neck, you probably don't have a large head, but if you have a longish neck and a largish head then the skull bones are probably filled with air to compensate. Throughout the animal kingdom, the most evolved shape of any animal's body tends to favour the most stable centre of gravity. This protects the stability of the spinal column, which in turn helps to safeguard all its functions. That is, until you decide to walk upright and become a human being.

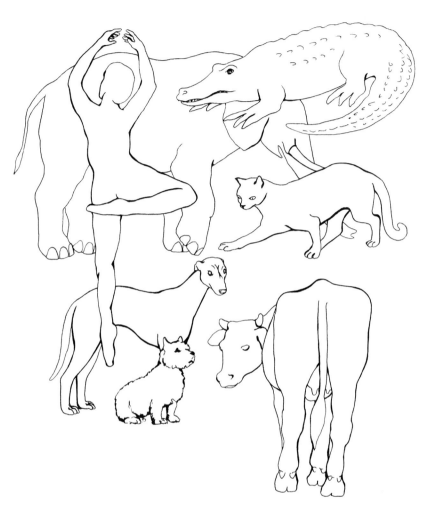

THE HUMAN BACK

The upright carriage of the human being is usually held responsible for all the things that go wrong with its spine. There's more to it than that. The spine evolved to house and protect the spinal cord, a long, closely knit bundle of nerve-fibres, which connects the brain – itself a network of nerves – directly to the rest of the body. The brain is the highest command centre for all the physiological processes which keep the body running. However, the brain has the capacity to generate thoughts, senses and emotions. These not only create our behaviour, they influence our physiology. Whether we are ambitious, susceptible to stress, an optimist or a pessimist, an introvert or an extrovert, open and loving or angry and rustrated, these mental states affect the function of all our organs, including the musculoskeletal system. Our entire self-carriage as human beings owes just as much to our individual mental configuration as it does to our evolutionary status.

The modern human body is unstable. That is, it's just about fine as long as it stands still over feet that are placed shoulder-width apart (even though this is no guarantee that it will not topple forwards or backwards). The moment a leg is lifted to take a step, the centre of gravity falls outside the body's frame and has to be re-established each time the weight is shifted from one foot to the other. Learning to walk on two legs is not only a question of developing a sense of balance, it also makes enormous demands on the strength and flexibility of the spinal column. Add to this the expectations, ambitions and social pressures which surround the human body as it grows from infancy to adulthood, and it makes just walking upright an almost Olympic achievement.

Nevertheless, as soon as we have mastered the art of walking, we immediately set out to find new challenges for the musculoskeletal system: we make our base areas smaller, our distance from the ground greater, our centres of gravity more unstable: we start to run, jump, try to stand on one leg, even on the point of one foot, or upside down, on our hands. As if this were not enough, we then do it all over again on moving objects, such as bicycles, motorbikes – and horses.

Mechanical devices used in sport – motor cars, bikes, cricket bats, golf clubs, skis – respond to the human operator in a predictable way. Their parameters of movement are predetermined because these are a product of the design. Not so with the horse. In equestrianism there are two sets of variables, the rider *and* the horse. There are two locomotor systems, each with a central axis full of nerves, and there are two separate command centres, which have their own thought processes, their own instincts for survival and their own mental priorities. Furthermore, the two spinal columns are not parallel, they meet at right angles: the vertical rider, whose centre of gravity now hangs off the end of his spurs, and the horizontal riding horse, who now finds *his* centre of gravity somewhere between his shoulderblades – and that's only while they're both standing still! When we consider the steps achieved by horse and rider combinations in any equestrian discipline, we can begin to understand the demands made on their individual senses of balance, their co-ordination, and their backs.

The back contains an information highway. The way this information is processed, through the relative position of the rider's back to that of the horse, is absolutely unique. Problems occur when for any reason this information becomes confused, because it automatically leads to loss of balance. Of course, this would not be so likely to happen if the horse, at least, had short, stocky legs, an altogether thicker neck, a much lower head carriage, and a good strong muscular tail – but then, who wants to ride a crocodile?

THE HORSE'S BACK

At some point in history, man looked at the shape of the horse's back, and decided to sit on it. It is, after all, a particularly inviting shape, a sensuous shape, a shape that is unique in the animal kingdom. Of

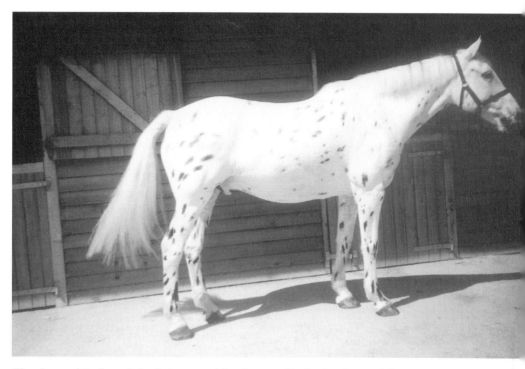

The shape of the horse's back is created fundamentally by the shape of the spine.

course, over the centuries selective breeding has modified it to suit the needs of specialized equestrian disciplines; but essentially it has retained its fundamental structure, which must have fascinated man right from the start: he didn't go to such lengths to change the ox – at least, not for the purpose of riding!

The shape of the horse's topline has come to be synonymous with all the qualities we associate with the horse itself: grace, nobility, strength, elevation and speed. These can be harnessed by man, just by the putting on of a saddle, or so it seems. Sitting on the back of a horse offers man the possibility of extending his physical or mental being beyond the capabilities of his own body. For athleticism, speed or simply companionship, the

horse's back offers all things to all people

The shape of the horse's back is created fundamentally by the shape of its spine, or more precisely by the shape of the bony extensions which radiate from the top and sides of the individual vertebrae. These are called spinous processes, and they are there for the purpose of attaching muscles and ligaments. The dimensions of the muscles, whether short and fat or long and spindly, depend on the calibre of the spinous processes. The height, angle and breadth of the spinous processes determine how much room there is for muscular development. The bony foundation is therefore directly responsible for the muscular contours of the back. This foundation varies greatly between horses of different breeds and, inevitably, between the types of horses used in different equestrian disciplines.

The spinous processes are highest at the withers and broadest at the loins. Breeding has produced a great many variations in both these areas of the back, from the high withers in the Thoroughbred, to almost no withers at all in some driving horses; from the slender loins of horses bred for speed, to the broad loins of those bred for strength. Between these two extremes, there are almost as many permutations as there are horses.

The withers and the loins form the boundaries of the saddle area. Their shape determines how much area of the back is available for the saddle, through their height at one end and their breadth at the other. There are spinous processes at the withers that extend so far in height along the topline that the saddle is constantly forced towards the unsupported part of the back, beyond the ribcage. There are vertical spinous processes that are so broad, together with horizontal spinous processes that are so narrow, that the only suitable saddle would have to combine an impossibly wide gullet, with a ridiculously small bearing surface. On the other hand, there are those horses that have such low spinous processes at the withers, and such broad spinous processes almost everywhere else, that it's really anybody's guess as to where the saddle should actually be.

The shape of the spine and its attendant

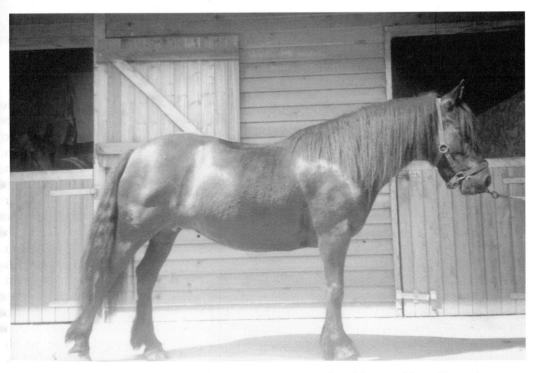

There are horses that have low dorsal spinous processes at the withers and broad lateral spinous processes almost everywhere else.

muscles have a direct effect on the way the limbs are used. There are back shapes that round easily and there are shapes that round only with great difficulty. Rounding the back enables the horse to bring his hind legs further underneath his body. This engages the muscle power in the hindquarters, which creates more momentum in the forwards movement without the horse's bodyweight being placed over the forelimbs. Good flexion of the hind limbs encourages the production of protective joint fluid; raising the forehand allows the forelimbs to follow through a more natural movement pattern, which reduces the effects of concussion. Therefore, horses that are unable or reluctant to round their backs – either because of their individual shape, or through injury or disease – are much more prone to degenerative processes in the joints of the hind limbs and forefeet than are horses that move fluently over their toplines. Conversely, painful concussion, which is symptomatic of degenerative joint disease, can be greatly relieved by paying constant attention to the suppleness and flexibility of the back.

Anatomically, the back is usually taken to mean the **thoracolumbar spine**, that is the part of the back from the highest point of the withers to the beginning of the quarters. However, this is rather like trying to describe the performance of a motor car just by talking about its drive shaft. The term thoracolumbar spine doesn't incorporate the shoulder-blades or the pelvis, which support the back at either end; it doesn't include the head and neck, with which the back has a reciprocal balancing function; nor does it include the tail, which is a reliable indicator of the back's comfort. It doesn't implicate the feet, or the shoes, over which the back is suspended, and it definitely doesn't include the saddle and the rider, which, however sympathetically placed, will always compromise the back's natural, physiological way of moving. So while 'thoracolumbar spine' might be synonymous with 'back', it is not the same as the horse's back!

To do the horse's back justice we really need a three-tier system of anatomy:

1. The regional anatomy.
2. The functional anatomy.
3. The combined functional anatomy of horse and rider.

The **regional anatomy** (the thoracolumbar spine proper) describes the bones of the spine (the vertebrae), the working parts (muscles, tendons and ligaments), the protective soft-tissue features (fascia and bursae), and the command elements (the nerves), as well as the nutritional supply and drainage system (the blood and lymph vessels). The **functional anatomy** includes all those structures most closely associated with the way in which the back works, namely the shoulder-blades, pelvis and ribcage, as well as the back's extensions at either end – the head and neck, and the tail. The **combined functional anatomy** describes the man-made frame within which the back has to move when the horse is ridden, namely the shoes, the bridle, the saddle, and the rider.

Whether it is viewed in the narrowest anatomical sense or in the broadest sense of a great, sporting horse-and-rider combination, the horse's back is a system of anatomical and mechanical complexity: on the one hand, it must have sufficient muscular softness to cushion the rider when moving slowly; on the other it must have enough skeletal rigidity for the rider to remain seated at speed. There are other animals whose backs are perhaps better suited to either one of these demands. Yet there are none that can achieve them both – and in such spectacular fashion – as the horse.

2 Anatomy

PRACTICAL ANATOMY

The horse's back was not originally constructed to carry significant weight on top of the spine. The fact that it can do so, even over obstacles or at great speed, is owed to the horse's unique anatomy, which gives its back a combination of elasticity and rigidity. However, in case we should be tempted to think otherwise, the features of the back that most enable us to sit on it evolved through physiological and behavioural necessity, not because they saw a saddle coming!

The back of the horse has to serve him at rest, steadily browsing with his weight mainly over the forehand, in flight, when his weight shifts in response to the terrain, and in the act of procreation, when the bodyweight is balanced over the quarters. For this reason, there are some parts of the back that need to be fixed and some parts that need to be flexed, depending on the situation. Areas of flexion always require great muscular control, and it is these areas that are particularly vulnerable in the ridden horse.

In wide, open spaces such as the horse's natural habitat, it is desirable to have a clear means of communication: visual signals that cannot be misinterpreted, even at a distance. The horse communicates by using his body. He can change the shape of his head by pricking or flattening his ears, or change the shape of his body by arching his neck, elevating the forehand, rounding or hollowing his back, raising or lowering his quarters, and lifting his tail. The topline of the horse, from the tip of the ears down to the last hairs on the tail, is a powerful means of expression: the intentions are clear, the signals are unmistakable. The art of riding simply choreographs the movements that are already in the horse's natural, postural repertoire.

We have probably all had the experience of riding a horse bareback, yet our more usual form of contact with the horse's back is through the medium of the saddle. It is not always easy, especially in competitive riding, to keep on reminding oneself that what is underneath the saddle is really flesh and blood. It is, after all, the saddle that is moulded to our backsides, not the horse. Like the favourite old armchair, it's often the well-worn saddle which gives the rider security, rather than the lean profile of the super-fit eventer, or the coiled-spring outline of a top-class showjumper. Nevertheless, whatever the shape of the back beneath the saddle, the anatomical building blocks are always the same. We need some idea of the consistency of these building blocks, as well as their function, before we can understand the strengths and weaknesses in the back's overall construction.

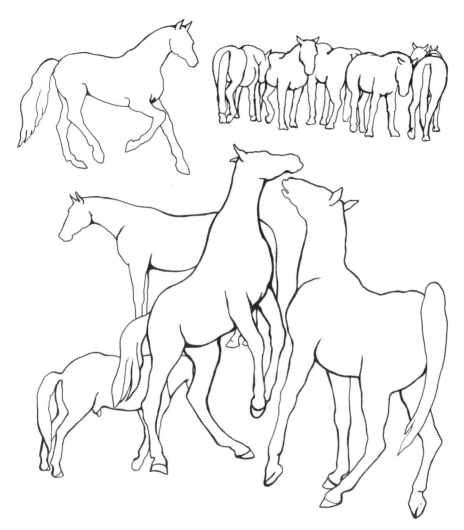

Bones

The spine is the solid core of the back. It is made up of individual vertebrae, which are essentially nothing more than a series of interlocking rings of bone. Each ring has a small indentation on either side, which, together with that of each neighbouring bone, form complete circular holes. These intervertebral holes are present all the way along the spine, and they allow the nerve fibres to leave the spinal cord at every intersection. The spine is really a very long, segmented tunnel, with service exits between each of the segments.

The rings of bone vary in size and thickness, and they have vertical and horizontal bony extensions, which are characteristic for the different sections of the back. The vertebrae in the neck are typically chunky, with short, but sturdy spinous processes, for the attachment of a

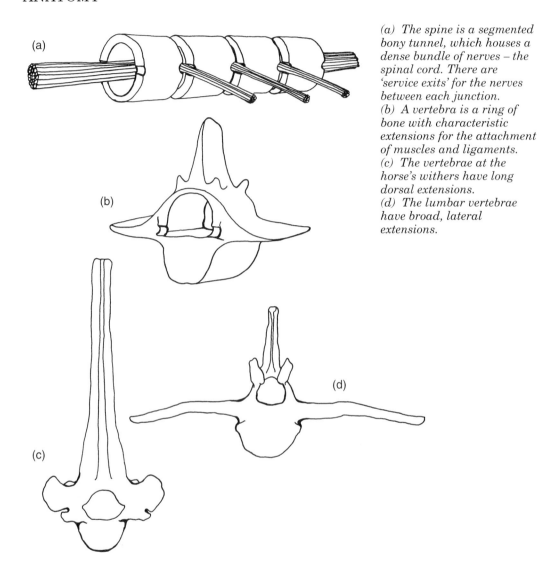

(a) *The spine is a segmented bony tunnel, which houses a dense bundle of nerves – the spinal cord. There are 'service exits' for the nerves between each junction.*
(b) *A vertebra is a ring of bone with characteristic extensions for the attachment of muscles and ligaments.*
(c) *The vertebrae at the horse's withers have long dorsal extensions.*
(d) *The lumbar vertebrae have broad, lateral extensions.*

layered system of muscles. This allows the neck bones to articulate in several directions. The vertebrae at the withers have long, dorsal spinous processes (in excess of 12in/30cm in some horses) which slope backwards and give the withers their characteristic shape. The spinous processes beneath the saddle are much smaller, positioned very close together, and nearly all vertical. In the loins the vertebrae are characterized by broad, transverse processes which make them look like aeroplanes. The profile of the quarters is created by the sacrum, a set of five vertebrae which are actually fused together. The large, horizontal process of the first element of the sacrum forms a connection with a similarly shaped part of the pelvis. Together they make a complete circle of bone – the pelvic girdle – of which the sacrum is a solid roof.

Ligaments

If the spine were a fixed rod, riding a horse would be like riding a penny-farthing bicycle or boneshaker! Because it is a slightly flexible, segmented tunnel there has to be some means of keeping it all together, and this must allow just the right amount of movement, without over-stretching. The vertebrae are literally strapped together by pieces of flat, slightly forgiving tissue, called ligaments. Ligaments have a certain amount of elasticity, but along the spine their role is to restrict movement rather than to facilitate it. The ligaments span the junctions between both the vertebral bodies and their spinous processes, creating a web-like corset of support for the spine. There are also long ligaments which run parallel to the length of the spine. These are attached to the tops of the spinous processes, as well as above and below the vertebral bodies, and they are more like tendons in their appearance. In particular the supraspinous ligament has consider-able tensile strength, rather like a nylon stocking when it is pulled taut. Unfortunately, like the nylon stocking when worn, the supraspinous ligament can develop holes if subjected to undue wear and tear.

Muscles

Like the ligaments, the muscles of the back fall into two categories: those that span short distances between neigh-bouring vertebrae, and those that extend over much of the length of the spine. Muscles contain fibres, which work on a ratchet system. When the muscle contracts, the 'teeth' of the fibres engage and the length of the muscle shortens. Depending on the stimulus, the muscle can then either relax, or it can continue to shorten. This process can be repeated until all the 'teeth' are engaged; the muscle has then reached the point of maximum contraction – it can't get any shorter. A muscle is very much like a sponge, both in the way in contracts and in the way it is fuelled. A sponge works only if it is compressed gently and then allowed to take up more water. If it is pressed to its smallest size and becomes totally dry, it loses its absorbing, sponge-like characteristics. This is important to remember when considering the back muscles of those horses that are continu-ally working in a high degree of collection.

Nerves

Imagine a microscopic, biological cell enlarged to the size of a football. Imagine it surrounded by thousands of extensions that give it the appearance of an Afro hair-style 10ft (3m) in diameter, and one single extension about the length of a football pitch. These are the relative dimensions of a single nerve-cell.

Nerves operate muscles: they are what every rider uses to make a horse go forwards, backwards, or up in the air. The body of every nerve-cell is often a very long way from the part that actually gives or receives information (the tip of the exten-sion), in some cases several feet. It is the long, single extensions that make up most of the spinal cord; the cell bodies are close

21

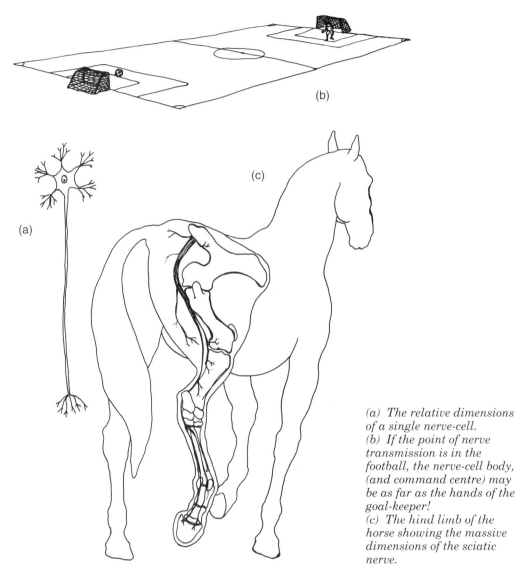

(a) *The relative dimensions of a single nerve-cell.*
(b) *If the point of nerve transmission is in the football, the nerve-cell body, (and command centre) may be as far as the hands of the goal-keeper!*
(c) *The hind limb of the horse showing the massive dimensions of the sciatic nerve.*

to connections in the brain. Information is passed to nerves in the rest of the body by means of 'junction-boxes' at the intervertebral holes. These nerves are also made of fibres which are bonded together and which may extend from the spinal junction right the way down a horse's hind leg: in a 17hh. horse that means several feet of nerve! If nerve-fibres are damaged, the repair has to be organized by the command centre in the cell body. It is often a long way to transport materials for repair down the whole length of a nerve-fibre, which is why nerves that have been compressed for a long time just don't get better: they have literally worn themselves out trying.

Nerve-fibres conduct their information using electrical impulses. The impulses travel at different speeds depending on the type of information to be relayed, from the very high-speed transmission of sensory signals to the relatively slow transmission of signals that stimulate muscle contraction. Nerves register changes in pressure, heat or vibration, they react to chemical changes in the surrounding tissue, and they monitor tension in joint capsules and tendons. They instruct muscle groups on the degree of stretch taking place in one individual muscle so that this can be supported by co-operating muscles, yet not interfered with by opposing groups of muscles. The nerves of the spinal cord make up an information super-highway, and we riders sit right on top of it.

Tendons, Fascia and Bursae

Picture a pork chop. A pork chop is a cross-section through one half of a pig's back. It is usually made of a right-angled piece of bone, part of the vertebra, and an area of meat. The meat is often divided into several parts, one large and one or two small. The meat, which is muscle, is pink; the dividing lines are white. Some of this white is fat, but the rest is a cross-section through the soft-tissue 'sleeves' that encase every muscle, separating it from its neighbours. At the end of each muscle body this tissue is drawn together to form powerful attachments to the skeleton.

In a limb, muscle power is transferred to the joints of the skeleton by means of tendons, dense bundles of high-tensile tissue originating from fibres close to the end of the muscle itself. Most of the muscles along the back span relatively short distances, allowing the backbones to move less than 1in (2.5cm) in any direction. These muscles don't need long tendons; their attachments to the skeleton tend to be flat structures of strong connective tissue. Some of these attachments, in life very white, smooth and glistening, spread over large areas of the body – for example, under the shoulder-blades or between the lower back and the abdominal muscles. Called fascia, this type of tissue forms a protective envelope around both muscles and their joints.

In machines, where moving parts glide backwards and forwards over fixed surfaces, there has to be some form of lubrication. This applies equally to tendons and ligaments, wherever they move over bones. To prevent fraying, the moving part is either kept moist by enclosing it in a self-lubricating sheath, or else the surface is cushioned by fluid-filled sacks called bursae. There are bursae along the topline of the horse to protect the supraspinous ligament as it passes over the top of the dorsal spinous processes. These bursae can become painfully inflamed when the horse is subjected to excessive bend over the neck and withers.

Blood and Lymph

Every living tissue needs energy. This energy comes from oxygen and nutrients which are delivered to the tissue via the bloodstream. No blood – no nutrients – no function: this is important to remember when considering some of the pressures exerted on the horse's back muscles by the saddle. Some types of tissue, like fat, have low energy requirements; other types, like muscles and nerves, have very high energy needs. Muscles have a means of extending their energy resources when oxygen is not immediately available, but even they cannot do this indefinitely.

Every cell in the body both contains and is surrounded by fluid. This fluid is not just a stagnant mass of water; it has special properties, which have to be carefully maintained, and it is responsible for the exchange of nutrients in and out of every cell. Any waste products of cell metabolism, which accumulate either when a cell dies or when it has been damaged, find their way out of the area initially in the extracellular fluid. This fluid is called lymph, and eventually it drains from large sections of the body into specific lymph channels.

REGIONAL ANATOMY

The spine is divided into sections according to the anatomical characteristics of the vertebrae. Although there are certain similarities between the last vertebra of one section and the first vertebra of the adjoining section, these divisions are far from arbitrary. They represent real functional units within the overall construction of the spine, and the junctions between these units are areas of increased vulnerability in the ridden horse. The sections of vertebrae are named for their situation in the body, and are often referred to by their anatomical initial: cervical (C) – neck; thoracic (T) – chest; lumbar (L) – loins. The exception is the sacrum (S), or os sacrum (holy bone), which is named after its role as a sacrificial offering in ancient fertility ceremonies. Within each of these sections, the individual vertebrae are numbered, so the third thoracic vertebra is described as T3. The parts of the spine which inevitably

come under the most scrutiny are the junctions between the individual sections. These are described by combining the two anatomical names together: cervicothoracic, thoracolumbar, and lumbosacral.

In the strictest definition, the term 'back' refers to the thoracolumbar spine. The first thoracic vertebra is situated between, and just in front of, the lowest part of the shoulder-blades. It is enclosed by some fairly 'heavy duty' muscles at the base of the neck, and is therefore impossible to feel and very difficult to treat. The first visible thoracic vertebrae are those at the withers, about T4 or T5. What we see are the tips of the dorsal spinous processes (DSPs), which in large horses can be over a foot (30cm) long. The height and slant of the DSPs in the thoracolumbar region give the back of the horse its characteristic shape, and their relative angles have important implications for the way the back is used under saddle. The DSPs slope backwards at the withers, but forwards at the loins. Those that are located directly underneath the rear half of the saddle are vertical, and altogether less massive than either of their neighbours. (The height of the lumbar DSPs is not as great as that of those at the withers, but their curvature is more pronounced). The gaps between the DSPs under the saddle are very small even in healthy horses. If, for any reason, these processes come so close together that they touch or even override each other, inflammation occurs. This is extremely painful, and the horse may adopt any number of strategies to avoid using this part of his back.

Apart from the distinctive shapes of its DSPs, the thoracolumbar spine is further characterized by being very well supported in one half of its length, and barely supported at all in the other half.

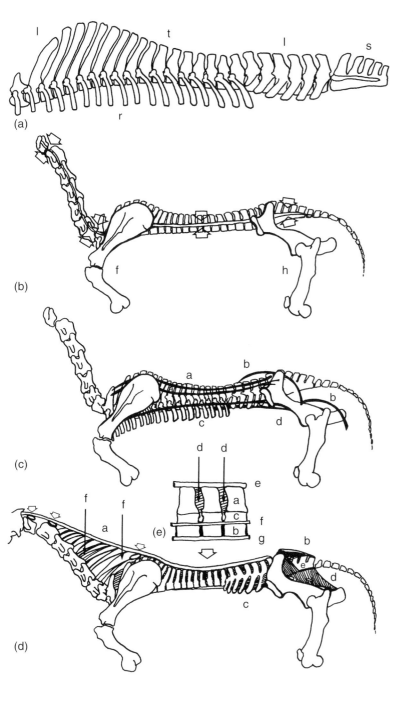

(a) The vertebrae of the horse's back: t, thoracic vertebrae; l, lumbar vertebrae; s, sacrum; r, ribs.

(b) The spinal column showing the position of the forelimbs (f) and hind limbs (h). Arrows mark the passage of the spinal cord.

c) A diagram of the large, superficial back muscles: a, the longissimus dorsi; b, the middle gluteal extending forwards into the gluteal 'tongue'; c, the iliocostalis; d, the iliopsoas muscles.

(d) Ligaments and bursae: a, the nuchal and supraspinous ligament; b, dorsal sacro-iliac ligament; c, intertransverse ligaments; d, sacrosciatic ligament; e, lateral sacro-iliac ligament; f, fan-like extensions of the nuchal ligament to the neck bones. Bursae are marked by small arrows.

e) A section of the back marked by the big arrow, showing the supporting ligaments of the vertebrae: a, dorsal spinous process; b, vertebral body; c, vertebral canal; d, interspinous ligaments; e, supraspinous ligament; f, dorsal longitudinal ligament; g, ventral longitudinal ligament.

The vertebrae of the thoracic spine are all attached to the ribs, which themselves are joined to the breastbone underneath the chest. This forms a solid skeletal cage. There is some movement in the ribs, as the ribcage is expanded by muscles for respiration but, apart from this, movement along the thoracic spine is minimal. After all, the rider is sitting immediately above the heart, the lungs, the diaphragm and some rather major blood vessels!

The lumbar spine begins where the ribcage ends, approximately at the back of the saddle. The vertebrae here have sizeable transverse processes, which provide areas of attachment for the long, powerful back muscles. There are also a pair of shorter muscles which run underneath the transverse processes, from just inside the ribcage to just inside the pelvis. However, apart from muscles and ligaments, there is nothing else between this part of the spine and the ground except for the horse's considerable digestive tract. The lumbar spine is literally suspended between the pelvic girdle at one end and the ribcage at the other.

The contours of the horse's back are familiar to every rider because that's what we put our saddles on. These contours are built up by muscles, which like the vertebrae are characteristic for this part of the back. At the deepest level, the spine is encased in a dense web of short muscles, which allows a small degree of movement between each of the vertebrae, but which is also responsible for its stability. Nerves exit the spinal cord between each of the vertebrae, so a high degree of movement along the spine would eventually result in the nerve-fibres being sawn through. The deep muscles of the thoracolumbar spine are covered by the long back muscles, the longissimus and the iliocostalis, which begin at the pelvis, extend along the loins parallel to the spine, pass across the top of the ribcage, and reach down to the base of the neck between the shoulder-blades. The longissimus muscle receives a great deal of attention in the treatment of back problems. However, the nerves that operate this muscle also have branches to all the deep back muscles, so that when a segment of the longissimus is in spasm – or worse still, paralysed – it is likely that the whole cross-section of the back on that side will be affected. Beneath the lumbar portion of the spine is a small group of muscles called the psoas or iliopsoas muscles. When the saddle, and then the rider's weight, are first placed on the top of the horse's back, these muscles immediately contract to stabilize the spine. Unfortunately, this also has the effect of stiffening the lumbar portion of the back and preventing the horse from suppling the quarters. The reason for allowing the horse sufficient time to warm up during ridden exercise, and *not* attempting to sit to the trot until the horse is ready, is to encourage the psoas muscles to relax, which enables the horse to work 'through' and then 'over' his back as a whole.

The muscles surrounding the thoracolumbar spine work co-operatively. They are responsible for supporting the spine as well as for moving the horse forwards. They provide both suspension and propulsion. If the quarters are fixed, they will lift the forehand; if the forehand is fixed, they will lift the quarters. If the muscles on one side of the spine are activated, we have flexion; if the muscles on both sides of the spine are used, we have roundness.

FUNCTIONAL ANATOMY

Roundness in the horse's back would not be very obvious to the onlooker if the curvature were not continued through the horse's neck and quarters. In functional terms it is really not possible to isolate the thoracolumbar spine: the *whole* spine is a dynamic unit, and it relies on a variety of non-thoracolumbar elements to operate successfully.

One of the most important structures, which influences the support of the horse's back, is the nuchal ligament. This is a long, almost tendon-like structure, which begins at the base of the horse's skull, crosses the ridge of the first and second neck vertebrae, and spans the crest of the neck to the withers. It is attached to the other neck vertebrae by a fan-shaped arrangement of elastic, soft-tissue extensions. From the withers the ligament is attached to the top surface of the dorsal spinous processes, and from here onwards it is known as the supraspinous ligament. It continues along the back until it reaches the last lumbar vertebrae. A new ligament begins over the top of the sacrum, leaving

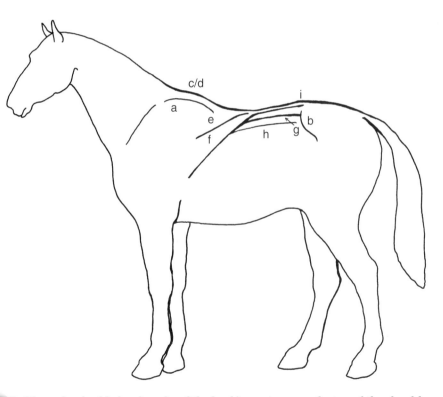

Visible and palpable landmarks of the back's anatomy: a, the top of the shoulder-blade (scapula); b, the point of the hip (tuber coxae); c/d, the dorsal spinous processes and the nuchal/supraspinous ligament; e, the trapezius muscle; f, the latissimus dorsi muscle; g, the longissimus dorsi muscle; h, the iliocostalis muscle; i, the lumbosacral junction.

27

a gap at the lumbosacral junction. When the neckbones are flexed the nuchal ligament is tensioned. This effect extends along the back as far as the lumbar spine, and is of great importance to the support of the lumbar back when the horse is working under saddle. If used correctly, it enables the back muscles to contribute more to propulsion rather than support.

The horse's abdomen contains the small intestine, the large intestine and the caecum. Together they have the dimensions of a bath tub. Imagine carrying all that round Badminton or Aintree! The horse therefore has powerful abdominal muscles to keep his digestive system in place. There are three layers of muscles which support the abdomen on either side, and one which supports it from underneath. However, keeping the gut in place is not the only function of these muscles, they also make a significant contribution to the support of the back. In the same way that a bow can be tensioned by drawing its string, pulling in the tummy muscles has the same effect on the spine. Horses that have been out of work for any length of time, and acquired 'pear-shaped' bellies, are often vulnerable in their backs because their abdominal muscles have lost their tone. Conversely, horses that hold themselves tightly in their bellies because of fear or stress, find it difficult to let their backs relax, and are therefore susceptible to the effects of concussion.

The nuchal/supraspinous ligament and the abdominal muscles combine to lift the horse's back by what is known as a 'double-drawstring' mechanism: one bow and string is the neckbones and the nuchal ligament proper; the other, inverted, is the lumbar spine and the abdominal muscles. Problems occur, both

in the neck and loins, when the horse is not able to use this mechanism to his best advantage, especially when carrying the weight of a rider. The exact degree of tension along the nuchal/supraspinous ligament depends on the weight of the head and length of the neck in relation to the length of the body. The horse knows best where to position his head and neck to make the most effective use of the nuchal ligament. The use of balancing aids should be carefully considered because they often interfere with this mechanism. Similarly, some horses naturally lift their abdominal muscles; others have to be encouraged to do so by the rider's legs. In riding, the legs activate the nerves to the muscles of the horse's belly, and this helps to increase the support of the back behind the saddle.

The thoracolumbar spine is fixed at one end to the shoulder-blades and at the other to the sacrum. The shoulder-blades are attached to the side of the ribcage by strong connective tissue called fascia, and the entire structure is suspended in a double sling of muscles, called the pectoral muscles. The last lumbar vertebra is linked to the sacrum mainly by muscles because the horse needs a high degree of flexibility at this junction (even if it's only for having a pee!). The sacrum, on the other hand, has large flat bony extensions which are literally stuck to similar-shaped elements of the pelvis. Although this is called the sacro-iliac *joint*, it is not a joint in the sense that an elbow or shoulder is. Movement between these two bones occurs only when there is some tearing of the connective tissue fibres. The sacro-iliac junction as a whole is encased in fascia and the powerful muscles of the quarters, which prevent the bones from being dislodged beyond the normal degree of tolerance. In the event of a slip or fall, these muscles immediately go into spasm, holding the sacro-iliac joint often at the very limit of this tolerance zone. In this way the organs within the pelvis are protected from injury, even though the skeletal imbalance is very uncomfortable, and remains so until it is realigned.

Along the course of the spine, there are hundreds of tiny joints which allow for movement between each of the vertebrae. However, apart from in the neck, this movement is minimal – in some places as little as a few millimeters. There is therefore no means of safeguarding the back against the effects of concussion, other than by maintaining the suppleness of the muscles, and the elasticity of the ligaments and fascia. In fact, there is a close correlation between the range of movement in the joints of the limbs and the 'well-sprungness' of the back. Jarr one and it is almost impossible not to jarr the other!

COMBINED FUNCTIONAL ANATOMY OF HORSE AND RIDER

There is one part of the horse's body where – in natural circumstances – very little extra weight is carried, and that is in the

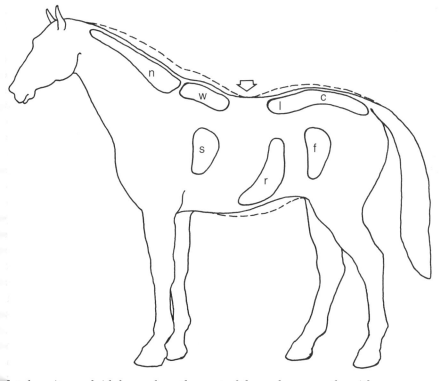

Fat deposits are laid down along the crest of the neck; n, over the withers; w, behind the shoulder-blades; s, over the loins and croup (l and c); over the ribs (r) and on the flanks (f). There is little room for excess weight to be carried in the saddle area (indicated by the arrow).

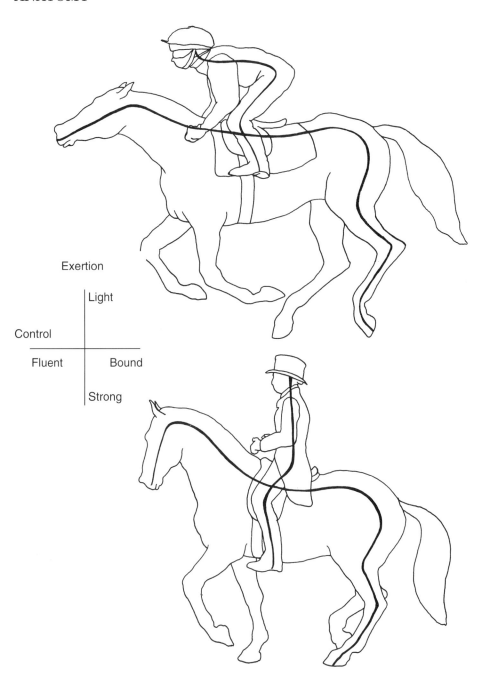

Exertion

Light

Control

Fluent   Bound

Strong

The choreographer Rudolf Laban devised a simple diagram to express the components of physical effort. This describes very aptly how the horse's back performs under the rider in different disciplines.

saddle area. Fat deposits are laid down across the withers, behind the shoulder-blades, over the sides of the ribcage, either side of the lumbar spine, as well as on the quarters: the horse may be carrying so much 'condition' that the spine itself appears sunken in a groove between two fatty bolsters, and this will certainly affect the fit of the saddle. Yet the amount of excess weight that actually exerts pressure on *top* of the thoracic spine is very small compared to the amount that can be carried on the neck and quarters, or even under the lumbar spine (as in the mare in foal). Therefore, by placing the equivalent of another 15 to 20 per cent of the horse's bodyweight directly on top of the thorax, we radically alter the demands on the horse's anatomy.

The horse's back is horizontal; the human back is vertical. The horse is an animal of flight and has an instinct to go forwards, which is reflected in the way he is built. The human back reflects the opposite movement, either upwards or downwards. Furthermore the human being differs from other animals in the development of the brain. The brain does not only control all the physical functions, it is also responsible for intellect. This means that, however much a movement may be part of a simple reflex response, it will nevertheless be strongly affected by the human being's personality. Human movements can never really be divorced from the mind that controls them. Depending on his mental constitution, a human can move with a lot of downward force, as if the whole world weighed heavily on his shoulders, or he can have a light, springy step as though he were walking on air. This applies just as much to the human who is sitting on the back of a horse. It is the human's state of mind

that determines how much downward, dominant, and potentially restrictive, pressure, we exert on the horse's back.

The combined anatomy of horse and rider cannot be described just in terms of changes to the individual centres of gravity. The combination is highly fluid, and depends on the interplay of forces that essentially act in two different directions, the horizontal and the vertical. These forces will not be the same from day to day, nor even from stride to stride – that's the challenge of riding. When they combine successfully there is harmony; when they

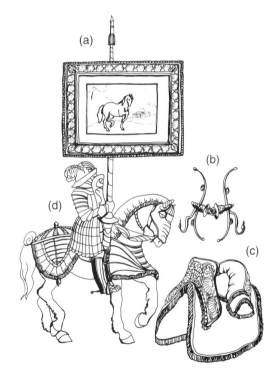

(a) Frames can enhance the content of a picture. Many different types of 'frame' have been used to enhance the performance of the horse: (b) A schooling (!) bit of antiquity (replete with spikes and rotating metal discs). (c) A saddle used by the Spanish Riding School. (d) A suit of armour.

clash, there is discord, and that is when backs develop problems.

As soon as man began to domesticate the horse, he also began to put a frame round him. Just keeping a horse in an enclosure is a kind of frame; and nowadays, with only a small amount of the countryside available for grazing and the need to rely much of the time on stabling, many horses are kept in frames within frames! Furthermore, we put shoes on their feet, bridles on their heads and saddles on their backs. These objects all contain elements that are as rigid as the fences around our paddocks or the walls around the stable. The shoes limit the natural expansion of the hoof capsule, the bit and bridle impose height and direction on the head and neck, and the saddle is strapped on top of those muscles that are supposed to carry the horse's body forwards. Even the most basic equipment for riding changes the horse's movements from the way he would perform them naturally. It creates a frame.

Picture-frames can enhance or detract, they can be simple or ornate. A heavy gilded frame can draw attention to a beautiful miniature, but a skimpy piece of plastic around a badly positioned subject can repel, even when there is nothing else to look at in the room. Throughout history,

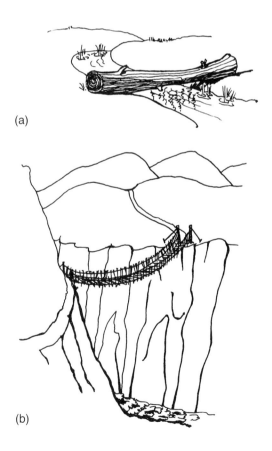

(a)

(b)

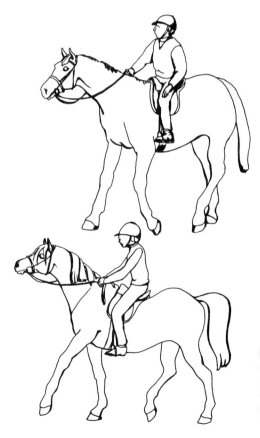

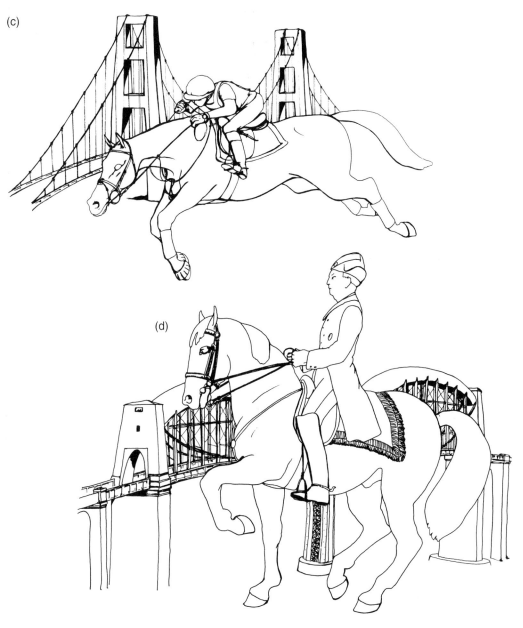

The horse's back is like a bridge. Without specific instructions from the rider, the horse may choose to use the rigid elements of his back, like (a) a single-beam bridge; or the soft-tissue elements, like (b) a rope-bridge. The combined use of all the back's elements give it the strength and elasticity of (c), a suspension bridge. When the horse achieves maximum collection, the interplay of the back's component parts is highly complex, like (d) the Royal Albert bridge over the river Tamar at Saltash, designed by I. K. Brunel.

33

horses have been contained in the riding equivalent of gilded frames: the baroque dressage horse wore convoluted curbs and chains; horses in Greek antiquity had bits with discs and spines; the medieval war horse carried the entire weight of a man in a suit of armour, on saddles built like howdahs. Yet these horses were no shrinking violets! Literature on the art of horsemanship through the ages has always emphasized the glories of the horse's self-carriage (whatever the severity of the training methods). Today's horse is almost naked by comparison, wearing lightweight materials such as aluminium, polyurethane, and the ubiquitous neoprene, yet these are by no means a guarantee that the horse will develop presence and self-carriage when ridden. The frame still has to complement the picture.

In previous centuries, training in the art of horsemanship was based on one type of horse for one type of discipline. Today there is a huge diversity in shapes of horse, and an incredible range of tasks that each shape might be asked to perform. For example, take the typical life of a horse bred through the centuries for racing, the Thoroughbred. It perhaps doesn't quite make the grade, so it is sold off, having trained and failed before most other breeds are even backed. It does a bit of hunting, has a couple of seasons point-to-pointing, and is sold, owing to circumstances, to become a riding-club horse. It is showjumped until the joints begin to look a bit suspect, and from there on becomes a dressage horse. Eventually it is retired from competition altogether, but to keep it from really getting stiff it goes hacking two or three times a week. This is a fairly standard chain of events for many such horses, but it is also *one* shape of horse and *one*

shape of back that in a single lifetime may have to fulfil half a dozen different expectations. It can be done, of course, but one has to take into account the strengths and weaknesses of the horse's shape as an individual. Nowadays there can be very few generalizations when it comes to training backs in the modern riding horse. Just look round any competition warm-up area and you will see as many shapes of horse as there are shapes of human being sitting on them.

Under a rider, the horse's back functions like a bridge; not just one kind of bridge, but any kind, depending on what the rider is wanting to do. A bridge is designed to span a low-lying area or obstacle, between two higher pieces of land. The simplest bridge might be a plank or tree-trunk across a stream: solid with a small degree of elasticity, but on the whole not very versatile. Another might be a rope-bridge across a ravine: highly flexible, but rather precarious. The spine of the horse is like the plank, spanning the distance between the forelimbs and the hind limbs. The back muscles, in their untrained and rather flaccid state, are like the rope-bridge. The horse carrying a rider on his back at walk and trot, with little contact on the bit, and no element of collection, can use his back like either one of these bridges. He only has to accommodate the extra weight of the rider, so he can use the rigidity of the spine or the elasticity of the muscles depending on the situation. Used in this way, the horse's back is enduring and low maintainance but not very versatile.

The suspension bridge, on the other hand, achieves a high degree of elasticity through the cables which suspend the platform from tall pillars at either end. This kind of bridge probably comes closest

34

to illustrating how the horse uses his back when trained primarily for speed, either racing, eventing, or hunting. These horses are not working in collection but need a high degree of flexibility in their backs especially across country. The pivotal points are the shoulder-blades and the pelvis, which are like the upright pillars of the suspension bridge; the back muscles are the cables lifting the spine from either end.

The advanced dressage horse or showjumper spends a great deal of his training with his back rounded in the highest degree of collection. This back is best described by Brunel's famous railway bridge over the river Tamar at Saltash. This construction combines features from all the other bridges: the single beam, the arched span, and the suspension bridge. For advanced movements like *passage* or *piaffe*, or for jumping large combination fences with precise stride lengths, the back has to have the maximum amount of stability whilst unfolding the greatest amount of elasticity to produce the greatest muscular strength from the most rounded muscular shape. Brunel's bridge was an extraordinary piece of engineering, and so are the backs of these horses.

A bridge allows free passage without hindering whatever is directly underneath it, such as a river or road. This is also true of the horse's back. Beneath the horse's body is the space occupied by the limbs. The greater the degree of lift in the back, the more the horse is able to bring his hind legs, unhindered, into the space under his belly. What is more, bridges also have to withstand the constant movement of traffic across them, including the weight and vibration caused by the movement. The horse's back is the same. It might be possible, for example, to drive a truck over a primitive rope-bridge, but probably not more than once! Every horse's back allows him to carry out the full spectrum of movements that he requires in his own natural environment. What it doesn't allow him to do, is to carry out repetitive and demanding movements without first being adequately prepared. When the hunt goes by, every horse can *passage* and *piaffe* with the best, but that doesn't mean to say they can do it for hours, or even want to. A flying change done once, out of curiosity or a bit of fun, never did any harm; but if it is repeated on a back that is not strong enough, you are likely to find the analagous truck at the bottom of the ravine!

History has given us blueprints for horse's backs which were bred for specific purposes: the draught horse, the medieval war horse, the baroque dressage model, the light carriage horse, and the racing Thoroughbred. A modern riding horse can combine elements of all these, but the kind of bridge you can build depends very much on the kind of shape you start off with.

3 Shapes

Compare a tractor to a racing car. They are both essentially single-seater vehicles with extremely powerful engines but they are very different in shape: the one would become pretty unstable at 200 miles (322km) per hour, and the other would not be much use ploughing a field. It all depends on how the power is distributed to the machine. Similarly there are shapes of horses that lend themselves naturally to certain disciplines, and there are other shapes that are extremely vulnerable unless the idiosyncrasies of their 'design' are taken into consideration.

The ten fundamental ingredients of the horse's shape are:

1. The length of the back compared to the length of the legs.
2. The height of the quarters in relation to the height of the withers.
3. The breadth of the back musculature from across the withers to across the quarters.
4. The length of the neck.
5. The weight of the head.
6. The angles of the limbs; in particular, the slope of the shoulder, the length and slope of the pastern, and the angle of the pelvis.
7. The extension of the gluteal muscles over the loins, called the gluteal tongue.
8. The definition of a 'second thigh'.
9. The depth and breadth of the horse's barrel.
10. The openness or uprightness of the hooves.

Stir these ingredients into a large melting pot, and you will end up with any one of the countless variations that represent today's modern competition horse. There are Warmbloods cross Thoroughbreds, Arabs cross cobs, Thoroughbreds cross Arabs, cobs cross Warmbloods; and they all come with their own special driving force, namely the mentality inherited from any one of the parental breeds. If you're lucky, you can get the best of both worlds; if you're unlucky, well . . .

Leaving aside the variations, let's consider four basic foundation shapes, and their possible implications for the back.

1.   BASIC SHAPE: ARAB

Very typical of the Arab is the dished back, and the natural inclination towards a high head and tail carriage. The back is relatively short; and although Arab breeders don't care to admit it, many Arabs do in fact have a croup that is as high if not higher than the withers. The hind legs are long, but the joints are often rather upright. The back should have a natural springiness, with a generous breadth of

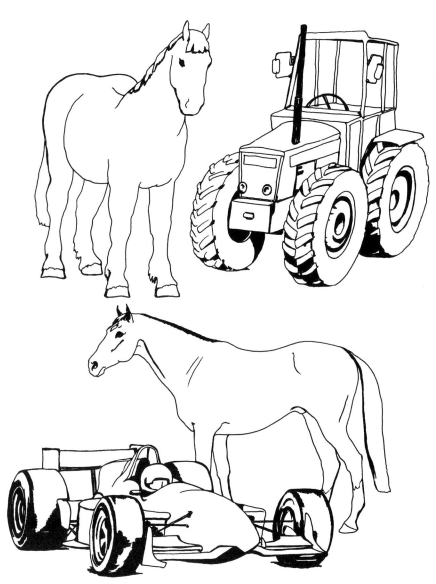

back musculature compared to the width of the chest. There is good support from the gluteal muscles which extend well over the pelvis into the lumbar region. The overall picture of an Arab should be one of lightness (or even, sometimes, light head-edness) and endurance. However, there is a great difference between dished and dippy. An Arab with a dippy back is almost certain to develop painful inflammation around the spinous processes in the mid-back region.

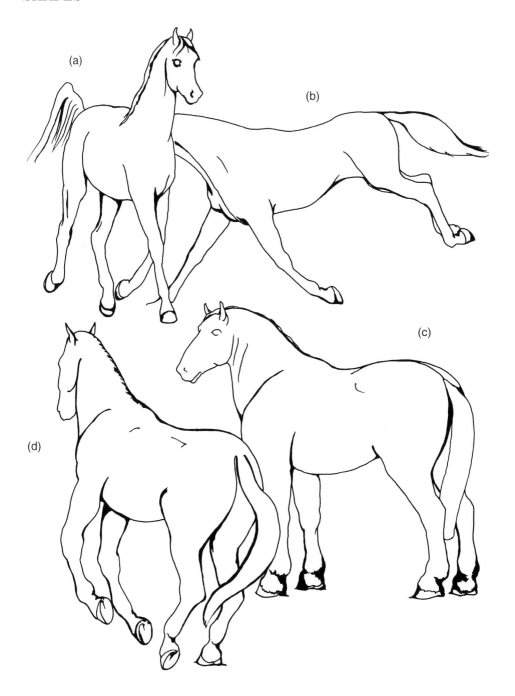

Four fundamental shapes of back: (a) the Arab; (b) the Thoroughbred;
(c) the cob; (d) the Warmblood.

2. BASIC SHAPE: THOROUGHBRED

There are many types of Thoroughbred, depending on the blood-line, but they all share certain musculoskeletal character- istics: high withers; long legs; long, sloping pasterns. The back length can be variable, but the breadth of muscle – particularly across the loins – is usually narrow for the overall build. There is often an accentuated slope to the pelvis, which contributes to the ground-covering and jumping ability of the hind limbs. The development of the gluteal muscles over the quarters, through race training, often gives the impression that Thorough- breds are croup high. At any rate, whether they are sprinters or stayers, Thorough- breds are bred for speed. Their build is designed to carry the whole body forwards under its own momentum. The loins are not well supported by the gluteal 'tongue', which means that the lumbosacral junc- tion is extremely vulnerable, especially if the pelvis is steeply angled. The long back muscles are often not broad enough to carry serious weight. The Thoroughbred back is a 'forward-thinking' back, and it really gets into trouble if it is subjected to the downwards force of a particularly dominant sort of rider.

3. BASIC SHAPE: COB

There is quite a variety of cobs, from com- mon drays to show cobs. However, think of a cob, and you will almost certainly think of roundness and stability. The wither profile is dominated by the chunky build of the shoulders. There is equal provision for muscle bulk over the shoulders and the quarters. The pelvis is

often steeply angled which gives the cob good jumping ability, yet the back is generously supported by the gluteal 'tongue' which makes its conformation reminiscent of the baroque dressage horse. This, together with a usually short, stocky neck, means that the cob is capable of positioning its bodyweight over the hind legs or thrusting the body forwards over the forehand. This has led to the use of the cob as a dual-purpose animal, for riding and for driving. Problems occur when cobs that are broken primarily to harness, and thus accustomed to throwing their weight for- wards, are suddenly turned into riding horses without any preparation. Their backs may be broad, but they are not necessarily strong under the additional and unfamiliar weight of a rider. Cobs with long backs particularly suffer from painful spinous process problems if they are not taught to use their backs differ- ently under saddle.

4. BASIC SHAPE: WARMBLOOD

The continental Warmblood is largely influenced by the Hanoverian breed. The outstanding feature of this type of horse is the stability of its back under saddle. The breadth of the back muscles, and their flatness over the pelvis, mean there are no awkward junctions – such as around the withers or the sacro-iliac joint – which are susceptible to strain through lack of muscular support. The overall build of the Warmblood's back gives its stride a natural elevation, which is often achieved in other models only through specialized training. However, even the Warmblood's back is not infallible. Their mentality is

39

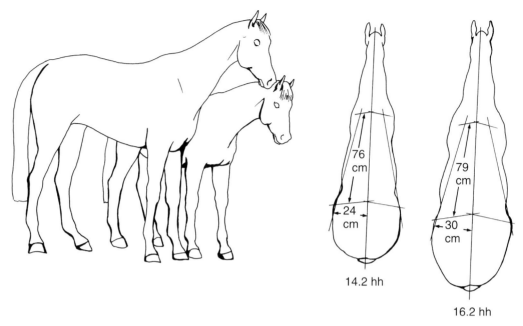

Measurements were taken from two horses of differing heights. Their back dimensions were almost identical.

more 'grounded' than other breeds, making them more suited to disciplines that require constant repetition of movements. Their stoicism in training often prevents the early recognition of ligament strain or muscle spasm, and they are often criticized for substandard performance when in reality they are suffering from an injury.

WEIGHT-CARRYING POTENTIAL

The shape of the horse's back is created by the skeleton, which provides places of attachment for the muscles, and by training, which increases muscle bulk by stimulating the blood circulation. Backs of horses are, however, extra-

ordinarily deceptive: the overall size of the horse has nothing to do with the strength or weight-carrying potential of his back. Probably the strongest back per cubic yard of horse actually belongs to the Shetland pony! For example, in one test measurements were taken from two backs: one belonged to a 16.2hh. Thoroughbred mare, the other to a 14.2hh. native pony cross Thoroughbred. Measurements were made from the tuber coxae (point of the hip) to the highest point of the sacrum, and from the tuber coxae to the highest point of the scapula (shoulder-blade). The measurements were identical. One would have assumed that the bigger horse could be ridden by a bigger person, yet the smaller horse was actually much better designed to cope with a heavier weight of rider.

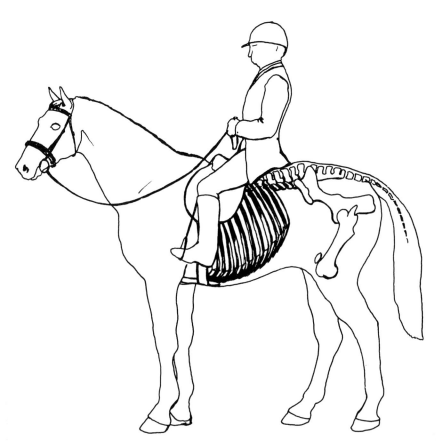

It is not necessarily the actual weight of the rider, but his position on the horse's back that causes problems, especially if he sits over the unsupported part of the horse's spine.

The amount of weight that a horse's back can support, therefore, depends on the shape of the horse *and* the shape of the rider, not just on the size of the entire horse. There are probably few real absolutes as far as rider weight is concerned. It is more a question of where and how that weight is distributed. The most stable part of the horse's back is over the ribcage because this is virtually an enclosed circle of bone and has little movement. On the other hand, the lumbar vertebrae are entirely dependent on muscles and soft tissue for support. If the saddle and the rider's weight rest on this part of the back, it makes it almost impossible for the back muscles to move fluently. The entire back mechanism becomes disabled. Riders that have long legs but ride with short stirrups are in danger of placing their bodyweight over the unsupported part of the back, and then it doesn't matter how heavy or light they are. In horses with high, and long, sloping

41

withers, and powerfully built shoulders, there is often no room for the saddle to rest in the correct position because the shoulders push it backwards over the loins. Such horses are not good weight-carriers, however big they may be.

If the eye is the window of the soul, then the horse's back is certainly a mirror of his well-being. The horse's back is not just a place to put a saddle; it's a complex machine and it's alive. It might have only one horse-power, and sometimes no brakes, but it has a reasonable top speed, does lots of miles to the gallon, and it even jumps obstacles. Unfortunately, you can never get hold of one that comes with a decent manual of instructions! It is therefore inevitable that the horse's back will need some servicing, however well we look after it.

4 Mis-Shapes ─────────

One of the most debated subjects in the whole of equestrianism is whether or not horses have bad backs. For some horsemen, a horse with a 'cold-back' is merely demonstrating eccentric behaviour; for others, every unexpected response is indicative of a back problem. For still more it's all a bit of a mystery, but they sign their horses up for the backman, anyway. Clinical conditions such as laminitis, degenerative joint disease, navicular syndrome or azoturia can be confirmed fairly easily by readily available diagnostic means, such as X-rays or blood-tests. Bad backs, however, are diagnostically both complex and expensive. Furthermore, the whole question as to whether or not the back is bad is often highly subjective. What is acceptable to one observer in a horse's way of going; may not be so to another: the only person who can really tell is the person sitting on the horse. There are many instances when a rider has felt there is something 'not quite right', only to be told to carry on regardless. It can be a costly error of judgement not least for the horse.

The main area of confusion is in the terminology. A variety of different expressions are used to describe what might turn out to be one and the same condition. Backs can be 'sore', they can be 'cold', they can be 'out'. They can have pain, they can have a problem. Or else one can get terribly technical and talk of subluxations and paravertebral reflexes, kyphosis and lordosis, ankylosis and spondylosis. All these terms are descriptive, but they do not really give the rider any information as to how the performance of his horse's back is impaired. In a lameness diagnosis, we expect to identify the area of the limb that is causing the problem, the type of tissue involved, tendon, joint, or muscle, and then decide whether it is a painful lameness or a mechanical one. The appropriate treatment depends on the accuracy of this information. Unfortunately, backs are often treated without any sort of information whatsoever, and one wonders why they don't get better! Methodical investigation is just as necessary for a back as it is for a front- or hind-limb lameness, with one small addendum: whereas the cause of a lameness can usually be identified independently of the rider, it is very important when diagnosing back disorders *not* to disregard the information given by the person in the 'driving seat', who may have experienced, at first hand, the very incident that precipitated the symptoms.

Back disorders fall into two categories:

1. Back pain.
2. Back problems.

Pain occurs whenever sensitive nerve-endings register chemical changes in surrounding tissue. Chemical signals are produced when there is damage. This might be the result of compression, heat, lack of blood supply, cold, or the introduction of incompatible chemicals through creams, lotions, or internal medication.

Different types of tissue have different densities of sensitive nerves, and not all pain messages reach the conscious part of the brain (the cerebral cortex). Furthermore, the perception of pain varies among horses just as it does among humans: there are horses that are 'thick-skinned', and those that are 'thin-skinned'; some that are naturally submissive and others that are rebellious. The quality and quantity of pain depends on the type of signals reaching the brain, and on the type of brain that receives the signals.

Back **problems**, on the other hand, do not have to be painful – at least not to begin with. They can be the result of a horse using his back inappropriately for the type of work he is doing, either through lack of training or lack of understanding. For example, a horse that has spent several years propelling himself forwards in a straight line along a race track, cannot be expected suddenly to round his back and keep his balance on circles in a small arena. Such a horse will certainly encounter problems, along with several misunderstandings; but they don't have to be pain-related, just brain-related!

Reluctance to let the back swing freely is, more often than not, initially a sign that there is a restriction somewhere else in the body. Foot balance, the choice of bit, sharp teeth, uneven contact on the reins, and saddle-fit, may all inhibit the horse from responding to the rider, from 'giving' his back. Eventually one of these will cause a chain reaction, which results in part of the back becoming painful. Very often the rider may already have felt an imbalance or resistance in the back, indicating the development of a problem. The important thing is to follow it up, *before* the problem turns to pain.

SOURCES OF BACK PAIN

Bones and Joints

Every horseman knows that the bones in the horse's feet and limbs can suffer from wear and tear. Ring-bone, side-bone, navicular syndrome, spavin, and so on; we all know in our heart-of-hearts that these conditions are caused, in no small part, by concussion, jarring, jumping on hard ground, excessive flexion of some joints without the necessary degree of suppleness in others – in general, 'the hammer, hammer, hammer, on the hard high road'. The horse's spine can suffer in much the same way. For example, riders will try to force compliance in the horse's back by using gadgets, which in fact do little more than impose massive restrictions on the neck vertebrae. If they are not allowed to move freely, joints between the neckbones will definitely show the same signs of wear and tear as joints in the horse's feet. Pain in the neck region affects the balance and security of the whole back.

Bones can be remodelled. Bones contain two types of cell, called osteoclasts and osteoblasts, which break down and rebuild bone substance in response to mechanical pressures. This is not just a process that happens during growth. It continues throughout life, adjusting the strength of the skeleton wherever it is needed. The most obvious example of remodelling is in fracture repair, but joints, intervertebral spaces, and dorsal spinous processes can ll be reshaped if the body feels that it must do so to protect its own interests. The remodelling process begins with a signal. This is most likely to be in the form of inflammation, which is the body's response to constant trauma. Initially, special cells produce anti-inflammatory substances to relieve the inflammation. It's only when this measure is not enough to withstand the insult that minerals are brought in as reinforcement.

However, the vertebrae have very specific shapes, with extensions in several directions for the attachment of ligaments and muscles, as well as indentations for the passage of nerve-fibres. The whole spine is surrounded by a closely inter-woven corset of short and long muscles through which are threaded hundreds of nerves; these nerves exit the spinal cord at every vertebral intersection. There really isn't much room for the remodelling of bones here, without encroaching on the space required by these vital, non-skeletal elements. Positions of the individual vertebrae are closely monitored by nerve relays. Extra mineral deposits can change the width of the intervertebral spaces and cause deviations in the angles of the verte-brae. This can seriously threaten the integrity of the spinal cord. For this reason such conditions are associated with very loud pain signals.

There are six painful conditions which affect the spine:

1. Narrowing of the intervertebral spaces.
2. Narrowing or even complete loss of the spaces between the dorsal spinous processes.
3. Fractures.
4. Spurs of bone, especially close to the roots of nerves.
5. Narrowing of the spaces between the lateral processes of the lumbar vertebrae.
6. Bridging underneath the bodies of the vertebrae (spondylitis).

Any of the above can result in an abnormal fixation of the spine (ankylosis). However, as with similar changes in the hocks or forefeet (spavin, or side-bone, for example), once the body has achieved adequate stability the process of mineral-ization stops and the pain begins to recede. Pain occurs only as long as the surrounding tissues are irritated by

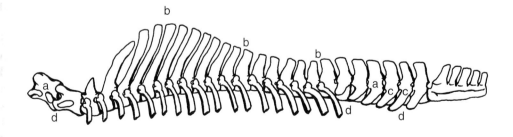

ainful conditions affecting the horse's spine are caused by: a, narrowing of the intervertebral spaces; b, crowding of the dorsal spinous processes; c, compression of adjacent transverse processes; d, extra bone formation underneath the vertebral bodies.

45

the rough surfaces of extra bone deposits, or when these deposits themselves are stressed.

Muscles and Nerves

Muscles are the servants of nerves. Any muscle dysfunction will be registered by its nerve, and any nerve dysfunction will have an effect on the performance of its muscle. Because muscles also contain sensitive nerves, which transmit pain signals to the brain, any condition that affects a muscle will invariably be painful.

For obvious reasons, muscle disorders are the commonest causes of back pain in horses. After all, muscles are what we put the saddle on, they carry us around the lanes and around the race track, they lift us over a hedge and ditch, or into the steps of a pirouette. In the human athlete, the muscles of the individual are at the command of that individual's brain. There is constant feedback between the brain and the body and, if used intelligently, the body's regulatory mechanisms can be encouraged to enhance its own performance. It's a closed system. For the equine athlete it's different. The equine body and brain might be relaying signals, but these are under the command of a quite separate individual. The moment we start to train a horse, we extend the chain of command from the horse's muscles to our own nervous system, and ultimately our own brain. *We* determine the overall length of the muscles, *we* influence the amount of circulation the muscles receive, and *we* decide the level of tone they are to achieve. (We even govern the muscles' basic nutrition by what we bring home from the feed store.) Yet the only reciprocal information our brains get from the

muscles and nerves of this separate individual is the optical appearance of the horse's body shape, and what can best be described as 'rider-feel'. It's not a very reliable way to practise biochemistry.

Muscle disorders in horses fall into two groups:

1. Those that develop through reduction in the nutritional supply
2. Those that develop through nutritional overload, or imbalance.

If you compress a muscle for any length of time, either by weight, (for example, with a saddle), by restricting its length so that it cannot relax between contractions, or by overstretching, you effectively cut off the muscle's blood supply. The reduction in circulation may be total or gradually cumulative, but the consequences are the same. The energy that fuels the process of contraction and relaxation runs out and the muscle can't unwind. Such an area of muscle is very vulnerable because it can no longer behave like a muscle. Eventually, compression of the muscle puts pressure on the motor nerve, squashing the nerve's protective sheath which also helps the nerve to transmit its signals. The result is silence. No message, no response. Except, that is, for pain signals because, in the meantime, lack of circulation has led to an accumulation of waste chemicals and these send warnings to the brain via the sensory nerve. Muscle spasm gives way to partial paralysis (paresis), which eventually gives way to total paralysis. It is not uncommon to find small sections of the horse's back muscles that are completely paralysed as the result of a slip or a fall. They might almost be considered insignificant if they did not have such a profound effect on the horse's athletic performance.

Muscles that are not used lose their bulk and their tone: they waste. This happens if they lose their nervous supply, but it also happens when there is loss of mobility in a joint. In this case the muscle/nerve combination is not paralysed, it is simply inactive. The blood supply is reduced because of the lack of activity. If the movement of any joint is reduced, the muscles that operate that joint become weaker.

High-performance muscles have high-performance nutritional needs. It could be said that all back muscles are high performance simply because horses are ridden! Certainly it is not only the high-performance horse that suffers from azoturia. In this disorder, the muscle function breaks down because the muscle fibre membranes become unstable. This is usually caused by an electrolyte imbalance. Enzymes from inside the muscle are leaked into the bloodstream, and these are measured both to confirm the initial diagnosis, and later to monitor recovery once the diet and exercise regimes have been adjusted. Azoturia, set-fast, and tying-up syndrome can produce a mixed bag of symptoms, from a slight tenderness over the loins, or a stiff and awkward gait at an unexpected point during exercise, to profuse sweating, rigid stance and obvious extreme pain. However, there are also incidents of acute back pain that produce symptoms of muscle damage similar to those of azoturia, even causing a rise in the same diagnostic enzymes. Owners are then persuaded to embark on an elaborate feeding system, which they religiously follow for years after the incident, when all the time the horse was suffering from an acute muscle injury that had nothing to do with tying-up at all. Cases of azoturia must be blood-tested regularly to support the diagnosis and assist the owner in what might be a very long period of convalescence for the horse (six months to a year or more).

Painful muscle conditions can affect any area of the horse's back, or any area of the horse for that matter. However there are some sites which, because of the nature of riding, are predisposed to pain. These are in the muscles located in the following five areas:

1. Either side of the withers, above the shoulder-blades.
2. Behind the shoulder-blades, under the points of the saddle-tree.
3. Either side of the last thoracic vertebrae, approximately under the rear third of the saddle-panel.
4. Either side of the thoracolumbar junction.
5. Either side of the lumbar spine.

Pain is most obviously detected in the superficial back muscles, that is in the trapezius muscles over the shoulders and the longissimus muscles either side of the thoracolumbar spine. The nerves to these muscles pass through several other muscle layers, and any superficial pain symptoms almost certainly involve these muscles too.

Muscles that are painful tighten up and become hard or flinching to the touch; they are usually described as being in spasm. If the spasm is not relieved, it gradually turns to paralysis. When a portion of muscle or a muscle group is out of action, other muscles take over their supporting or dynamic function. Because these muscles will try to fulfil a task for which they were not designed, they become overloaded and subject to stress. This in turn causes new areas of spasm. There is a secondary row of painful sites along the horse's body, which is in close proximity to

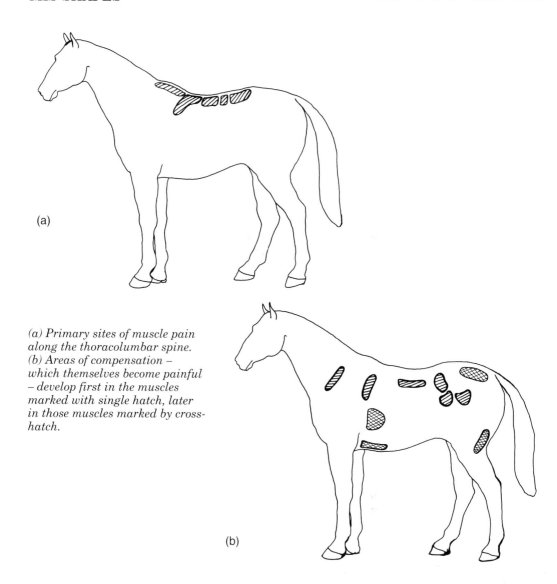

(a)

(a) Primary sites of muscle pain along the thoracolumbar spine.
(b) Areas of compensation – which themselves become painful – develop first in the muscles marked with single hatch, later in those muscles marked by cross-hatch.

(b)

the back and almost diagnostic of long-standing, deep-seated back pain. These muscle sites are found in four main areas:

1. In front of the shoulder-blade often in the mid-third of the subclavius and supraspinatus muscles.
2. Behind the shoulder-blade often at the same level as in 1. above, at the meeting point of the latissimus dorsi and triceps muscles.
3. In front of the tuber coxae (point of the hip) at the insertion of the iliocostalis muscle, or one 'hand' lower at the insertion of the oblique abdominal muscles.

48

4. In the quadriceps muscles below the hip joint.

Tendons, Ligaments and Fascia

Corsets, liberty bodices and body-stockings are made of strong, elasticated material, reinforced, and laced up if necessary. They are used to retain various parts of the body that might otherwise billow out into ill-defined shapes. Nature's way of doing the same is to use semi-elastic, immensely strong connective tissue, either in the form of dense bundles, such as tendons, short straps, such as ligaments, or broad, flat sheets called fascia. These structures have to be taut but pliable, rather like the leather suspension-straps in old carriages: to the body they fulfil a very similar function.

When ligaments and tendons develop holes, are overstretched or snap completely, they cause the same sort of imbalance that would occur in a carriage with faulty suspension. Things start to rub against each other which shouldn't, and this can be extremely painful. The entire bony tunnel of the spine, through which the nerves of the spinal cord pass, is held together by ligaments. Visualize the sudden snapping of the suspension on one side of a two-wheel carriage, and it will give you some idea of what it is like when a ligament tears in the horse's back. It's a nasty injury, to say the least, but one that can happen just by the horse's stepping awkwardly into a rutted track, or off a pavement curb, or even getting cast in the box. It has even been known to happen as a result of back manipulation.

Fibres of the supraspinous ligament – which runs along the top of the dorsal spinous processes – can tear just like the fibres in the tendons of the horse's lower limb. The injury is accompanied by the same sort of oedema and haemorrhaging that is found in tendon injuries. Diagnosis is made by ultrasound scan.

Fascia encloses broad areas of the body like a body-stocking. The purpose is to hold functional groups of muscles and joints in position – around the lumbar spine or over the hip joint, for example. Any trauma that sends a group of muscles into spasm, such as, landing wrongly after a jump, usually involves the fascia in that area, too. It may well be only the fascia that is left holding the joint at the very limit of its normal range of movement. Unfortunately, this creates areas of stress around the joint in other directions. The result is a loss of suppleness in all the surrounding muscles.

Injuries to tendons, ligaments and fascia tend to cause pain in the very structures they are meant to protect:

1. In nerves at the intervertebral junctions.
2. In joints, especially at the lumbosacral junction and the sacro-iliac joint.
3. In the sensitive tissue over the dorsal spinous processes.

Skin, Hair and Blood Supply

Watch five minutes of any television commercials, and you are bound to see an advertisement for a skin-care product or a shampoo. Whether they go on the hair, the face, or anywhere else on the body, we are fairly inundated with substances that are designed to make us appear to glow radiant with health. However, we all know that you can't really stick health on from the outside, and the same goes for the horse. The horse's coat and skin are the most significant indicators of his health, and this is particularly so along the back.

The skin is an organ, just like the heart or the stomach are organs. It has a metabolism of its own, it will permit some substances to pass and not others, it is sensitive to a great many different influences, and it has intelligence! The skin is made up of several layers of cells, the most superficial of which become hardened as they die off and are eventually sloughed. Embedded in the skin are the hairs, as well as different kinds of glands, which release moisture and oils onto the skin's surface, to cool the body and waterproof the coat. How does the skin know when to do these things? How does it know when it's hot, when it's cold, when to accept pressure, when pressure is harmful? How can it tell the difference between a butterfly and any other kind of fly? Because it's wired. The skin is thick with sensors, specialist nerve-cells that have evolved to interpret different kinds of mechanical and thermal influences and, of course, to conduct signals of pain. Nothing touches a single hair without causing an electrical impulse to be sent along a sensitive nerve-fibre to relay stations in the spinal cord and, if the message is serious enough, ultimately to the brain. When we sit on the back of a horse, we do so by kind permission of the skin.

Human beings are used to wearing clothes. The human skin learns at an early age to tolerate the feel and weight of different garments, as well as items of jewellery and spectacles or contact lenses. The horse learns to accept the pressure of a saddle, but in doing so he is entrusting a very vulnerable part of his body to his human handler, namely his back. In the wild, the back of the horse is the one part he can't defend against predators. Yet we expect him to wear numnahs, saddles and rugs of various thicknesses and materials, and to be totally at ease with them. The horse has to trust his human, and so does his skin.

The skin is not a barrier, it's a mediator. It interprets conditions in the environment for the body inside, and it reflects to the outside world how well that body is able to cope with those conditions. For example, a smooth, shiny coat lying on unblemished skin says to the outside world that its body is in harmony with the forces in its environment. A dull, staring coat, on a dry, flaky skin, is a body surface that is under attack from the environment and that lacks the necessary resources to withstand the challenge.

The challenges to the skin on the horse's back are enormous, especially when you consider that skin was never designed for the amount of pressure and abrasion that occurs under the weight of a saddle and rider. Then there are the surcingles, driving-harness straps, and anti-cast rollers which a horse may wear for several hours, and even in bed! They all have consequences for the healthy appearance of the skin and the hair along the back.

Changes that you might see, especially in the saddle area of the back are:

• Patches of broken hairs.
• Hair loss.
• White hairs.
• Thickened skin with sparse hair growth or no hairs at all.
• Raised, circumscribed areas with or without reddening or heat.
• Holes! That is, the surface of the skin

is actually broken and there is clear lymph fluid or blood visible.

Skin that is constantly being rubbed will try to withstand the insult by increasing the depth of the horny superficial layer of cells over the skin's surface. However, if the thickness of the skin increases, the blood supply to the hair follicles is reduced, and the hairs can be more easily damaged. Hairs that regrow after there has been a prolonged mechanical insult will usually be white because they lack the pigment provided by the blood supply.

The skin is a messenger: whenever it feels threatened it passes on the information to the underlying tissues, which include muscles. There are many types of therapy which use the skin to promote feelings of well-being in the body, so we can be fairly certain that negative sensations on the skin produce feelings of ill health. If the skin twitches uncomfortably, so do the muscles underneath, and that is not a very good preparation for putting on the saddle, let alone riding.

When it comes to the horse's back, if hairs are broken, or the skin is flaky, or there is any sort of exudate there will definitely be a change in the blood circulation to that area, either too much or too little. Once the blood supply becomes disturbed, waste products of the skin's metabolism collect, but they cannot be drained. The skin sensors register the change in chemical balance and begin to send out warning signals. The muscles beneath the affected area will always be influenced by a pain response in the skin, even if it is manifest only as a slight sensitivity. It may be just enough to stop a horse working really fluently through his back.

It is good to be really critical about even the smallest pimple appearing on the horse's back, especially if you want to sit on it, because:

• A glossy coat means a balanced blood supply and therefore a musculoskeletal system that is comfortable.
• Changes in the coat indicate changes to the skin's blood supply and very often a musculoskeletal system that is in need of comfort.

CAUSES OF BACK PROBLEMS

A problem is a difficulty which has to be overcome. It is something that is difficult to understand and that requires additional information or an increased level of understanding in order to come up with a solution. Unlike back pain, which already indicates that certain types of tissue are being threatened, back problems are simply an inability to use the back in a way that is indicated by the rider (or driver).

In any riding or driving career, a horse has to learn to go forwards, sideways, backwards and, in the case of jumping, also to clear obstacles. The horse is quite capable of doing these things by himself; but the point, as far as backs are concerned, is that he has to do them on command, carrying the weight of a rider, or having the restriction of a harness and vehicle. Commands are given by activating certain reflexes in the horse's body. Apart from verbal encouragement, the rider's legs and seat activate nerve-endings between the ribs and along the back which cause the horse to flex the back muscles, extend a forelimb, lift the belly, and engage the hind limbs. Yet what if the horse can't respond to these commands?

51

What if, for example, the saddle is too tight, or the foot balance is incorrect, or he is frightened of going forwards onto the bit because his teeth are sharp? Or he can manage one bend of his body but not the other because his pelvis is tilted, or even simply because he doesn't understand the command in the first place? What if the nerve-ending under the rider's left calf is telling the horse to go forwards while the mouth is telling him to stop because the rider's hand is unsympathetic? Soften the hand, balance the feet, rasp the teeth, adjust the pelvis, widen the saddle, and there is no reason why the back should not respond easily and accurately to the rider's aids. Back problems become painful – there is no doubt about that. However, in the first instance they are a symptom of difficulty and the cause is usually not in the back at all.

Lameness

Imagine a table, plain, rectangular and four-legged, but with one leg shorter than the other three. Instead of propping up the shortened leg, imagine insisting it always touches the ground, for example by putting a weight on top of it. If this is done over a long period of time, the top of the table will eventually become distorted and warped. Very much the same thing happens to the horse's back. Like the table, the horse's back is supported at each corner by a limb. However these limbs are attached not by joints but by very strong, connective tissue. The so-called sacro-iliac 'joint' is formed from two opposing, flat pieces of bone, which are virtually glued together; it's more of a join than a joint! The shoulder-blade is attached to the chest wall by fascia, and moved backwards

and forwards by muscles; there are no joints here either. When a horse stumbles, trips, lands awkwardly over a jump, puts his foot on a stone, receives a kick to a limb, or is involved in any one of the other countless scenarios which might lead to lameness, he tightens up the muscles on that limb to guard it against further pain: you or I would do just the same. This effectively makes one limb shorter than the other three. For a couple of days this will be of no consequence. Yet, very often, lamenesses can take weeks or months to resolve.

In order to keep his balance, the horse begins to tighten up an area of his back, usually on the side diagonally opposed to the injured limb. This restriction often remains after the injury has healed, preventing the horse from regaining his natural fluency and even predisposing the limb to further trauma.

In degenerative joint disease, or osteoarthritis, the onset of lameness is usually gradual. At first it is an almost imperceptible shortening of the stride length, in one leg and then the other, as the horse tries to avoid the precise movement of the joint which causes him pain. As the disease progresses, the muscles in the limb are no longer able to protect the joint from concussion, and the back muscles take over. If a forelimb is sore, the compensation occurs in the lumbar muscles on the opposite side of the spine. If a hind limb is affected, the compensation occurs over the opposite shoulder-blade. Initially this may be felt by the rider simply as a stronger trot stride on one diagonal, rather than a lameness. However, the cross-over point between the painful limb and the area of compensation is in the mid-back. It is not unusual to find that horses that have osteoarthritic changes in their hocks or front feet, often have secondary inflammation of the spinous processes in the mid-back as well.

Shoes

Have you ever been a tourist in any city and 'done' all the famous sights – the shops, museums and churches – and walked miles along hot, dusty pavements so that at the end of the day you're only too pleased to be able to sit down in the hotel, kick off your shoes, and put your feet up for five minutes? It's OK for us, we *can* take our shoes off, and any other restrictive clothing for that matter. There are jobs, too, where you might be on your feet all day and eventually your back starts to ache, but at least we can do something about it. What about the horse? What if his shoes don't quite fit him properly, or his feet are not quite in balance? This doesn't necessarily mean you have a bad farrier. It can happen as the horse becomes due for shoeing, for example, or when the kind of work he is doing encourages more growth in one part of the hoof wall than in another. Nevertheless, the horse is attached to his shoes twenty-four hours a day, even when he's lying down. If he has been competing all day, his feet are going to be tired just as yours or mine would be. If the shoes don't allow the hoof capsule sufficient room to expand and relax, the muscles in the limbs begin to tighten, and this eventually transfers itself to the muscles in the back. If the horse is uncomfortable *for any reason* on the feet, front or back, his response is to tighten up the back muscles, particularly those in the loins. By doing this he is trying to relieve the concussion. The problem is that this only makes his strides shorter, and actually increases the discomfort in the feet.

Until quite recently, it was generally taken for granted that most back problems were in fact caused by problems in the horse's feet. Even though we are now able to analyse the horse's back in greater detail thanks to improvements in diagnostic imaging techniques, there is still a great deal of truth in this assertion. The horse's back should swing freely, at walk, trot and canter, with or without a rider. If, every time your foot touches the ground, it jarrs the rest of your body (in trot, that might be sixty times per minute) your body will come to anticipate each moment of impact. The first symptom of uncomfortable feet is therefore loss of fluent movement. Conversely, it is amazing how quickly a horse is prepared to soften his back once his feet are comfortable again.

Saddles

Unfortunately, the same cannot be said of problems that develop through ill-fitting saddles. At the very worst, a saddle can be an instrument of torture, inflicting great pain and causing significant tissue damage to the back of the horse. However, in the majority of cases, the saddle will be only just that bit too narrow, or just a little out of balance: restrictive enough to prevent the muscles receiving adequate circulation during exercise, without actually causing pain. Far from being able to develop in response to training, the muscles under the saddle begin to waste. The horse starts to compensate by using a second 'tier' of muscles in front of the shoulders and below the points of the hip. If the muscle wastage is severe, the saddle eventually rests on exposed nerve-endings, which makes the back very tender indeed. The horse acquires a shorter, choppier stride and becomes heavy on the forehand as he gradually loses the ability to lift the forelimbs off the ground. The solution is to provide a wider-fitting saddle. However, a saddle needs something to rest on, and if the muscles have wasted, it can be a problem to recreate an area of back where there is none! Redeveloping back muscles that have wasted as a result of compression by the saddle is labour intensive, because it often involves re-educating the whole horse.

Teeth

In the wild, horses have access to a wide variety of vegetation, which not only provides a broad nutritional base but a great many different textures. They grind their teeth down naturally on coarse stems, and rougher grasses; no one comes round to them twice a year with a tooth rasp! Modern horse husbandry provides only a selected type of grazing and, combined with the use of energy-dense diets, makes it almost obligatory to have the horse's teeth rasped at regular intervals.

In addition, the head shapes of the domestic horse differ considerably from those of their wild counterparts: compare the latter with the short chunky head of some Arab lines and the long, narrow face of the Thoroughbred. If the teeth are not ground down by natural wear or rasping, the molars and premolars develop sharp points, which, especially in fine heads, very quickly catch on the inside of the

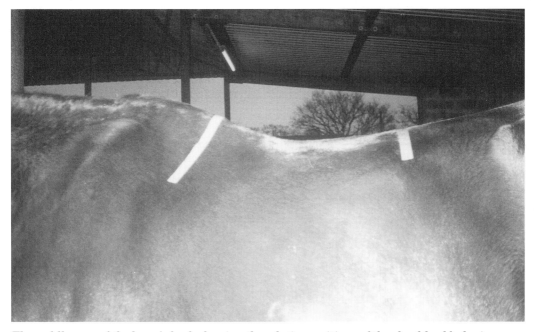

The saddle area of the horse's back showing the relative positions of the shoulder-blades in front and the unsupported lumbar spine beyond the rib-cage.

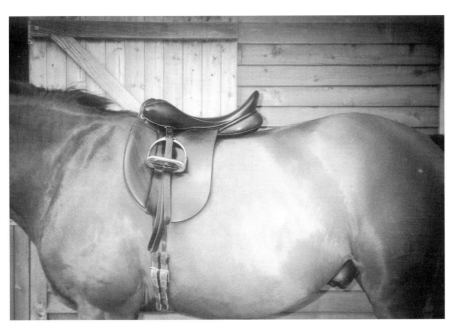

A saddle placed too far forward over the shoulder-blade.

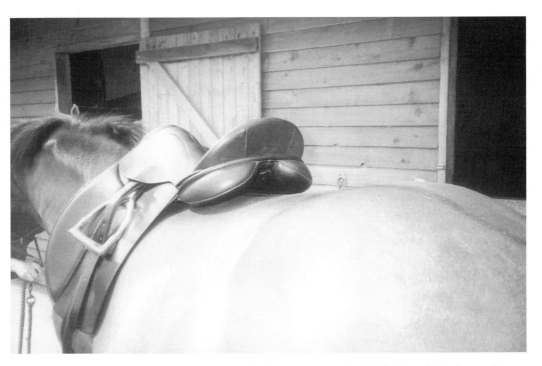

A saddle which moves too freely in the rear third, creating tension in the horse's back muscles.

cheeks. The horse may not actually drop his food, but he may nevertheless find it uncomfortable to relax his lower jaw to the pressure of the bit. The top jaw is wider than the lower jaw, so the only way the horse can stop the sharp upper back teeth from cutting the inside of the mouth cavity, is to set the bottom jaw. If the lower jaw is locked, then so are the muscles around the poll. Suppleness at the poll is essential to the suppleness of the back; you can't have one without the other. A horse that is uncomfortable in his mouth might as well have a brick wall in front of him; his movements become stilted and hesitant, and so does his back. The rider, however, will often feel a resistance in the horse behind the saddle, when in reality the cause of the problem is in front of his hands.

Behaviour

Horses are born to go forwards. They are, by nature, animals of flight, and it is their ability to go forwards with grace and power that attracts us to them. We associate the back muscles with forward movement, that is, when the quarters of the horse are stabilized the back muscles will lift the forehand off the ground. However, the reverse is also true, namely that when the forehand is fixed, the back muscles will lift the quarters, inevitably making it easier for the horse to go backwards. All movement sequences are reinforced by constant practice, and they are stored in a part of the brain called the cerebellum. Running backwards is no exception. In the face of danger, a horse's instinct should make him go forwards: even if, in actual fact, he spins round, this is still a forwards movement. Responding

to fear or uncertainty by running backwards is an aberation of the horse's most basic instinct, and horses that do this are profoundly disturbed and potentially dangerous. Their backs, which have actually rehearsed and stored the data for running backwards, are problem backs indeed!

Luckily, there are not that many horses that totally lose their natural instinct for forward movement. Those that do have certainly experienced a major physical or mental trauma, which often causes them to become withdrawn and expressionless. However, there *are* many horses that are ridden in a particularly restrictive manner, and that suffer from lack of impulsion as a consequence. This is reflected in their loss of self-carriage, lack of expression in their action, and absence of movement in their backs.

The way a horse moves depends on his personality. There are horses that come out of the stable ready to take on the world, there are others that are always in a hurry to get somewhere; some are just very businesslike, and others are just not very brave at all. There are horses that will go in front, there are those that would rather go behind. Just as with humans, there are leaders and there are followers. The horse that marches forwards with great determination will have a different tone to the back muscles than a horse that creeps along, hoping that no one will ask him to do anything difficult. The sheer anxiety of such an individual is enough to shut down the blood supply to his back, and leave his muscles thin and cold. In both types of horse it is essential that the rider allows and encourages forward movement, to maintain correct muscle development in the confident horse, and to give confidence through improved muscle development in the nervous horse.

The horse's back is like a musical instrument: it will play whatever tune the rider wishes, loudly, softly, liltingly or stiffly. If the rider is uneven, cramped, or hesitant, the 'instrument' will reflect this. It can also be played in tune, or out of tune. A back that is hollow is definitely a back that hasn't been tuned properly. Instead of round, well-formed sounds that harmonize, the notes will be brittle and just a little off-key. Unlike horses with back **pain**, those with back **problems** are often ones that just need playing in tune.

5 Diagnosis and Therapy

If a car has been involved in a collision, either with another car or a solid object, there is always the possibility that the frame has been bent. Incidents like clipping the pavement with a wheel, or driving over a pothole, can be enough to distort a small part of the chassis and leave the car difficult to steer. Just think how many 'collisions' a horse can expect in the course of a lifetime. They may be as trivial as two or three horses colliding as they all try to get through the same gateway at once, or as serious as taking a crashing fall at Aintree: collisions of any sort can jar the skeletal frame of the horse, overstretching ligaments or fascia and sending muscles into spasm. Muscle spasm occurs to protect joints from dislocation, and prevent damage to sensitive organs inside the body. However, muscles remain in spasm until they are actively released, which means the horse's frame is no longer symmetrical: in effect its chassis is bent.

Symptoms of acute pain are normally easy to recognize because there is a spontaneous reaction from the horse when we touch any area that hurts. Back disorders are often not like that. Structures that are jarred and misaligned are usually deep-seated and covered by superficial muscles. The presenting area of spasm on the surface of the back may only be the size of a walnut. In a 16hh. horse, such a place can go unnoticed until it affects the balance of other parts of the body. The horse may just be a little grumpy when saddled or worked, perhaps fidgety, or unresponsive to the rider's leg aid on one side. More often than not, these symptoms are put down to the horse's having an off day. It's only when they persist over several days or weeks that the possibility of a back disorder is considered. By this time, an incident that might provide clues as to the nature of the injury has been forgotten, and the grand debate begins as to whether or not it really is the horse's back at all.

For this reason, here is a checklist of typical incidents that can cause back disorders in the horse:

• Losing a foothold on a slippery surface, such as mud, tarmac, even some types of arena surface.
• Catching the point of the hip (tuber coxae) on a door-frame or gate-post.
• Pulling back on a lead-rope when tied up, especially if the neck is caught under the rope.
• Getting cast in the box.
• Putting a leg through a gate.
• Any kind of fall, tipping over back-

58

vards, landing upside down over a fence,
slipping full length sidewards.
• A sudden change of going, for example,
from tarmac to deep mud.
• Stepping off a pavement.
• A shunt from behind, for example, by a
vehicle or another horse.
• Catching a pole between the legs when
jumping.
Accidents in a horse-box or trailer.
Panic reactions.

The above situations are not freak accidents: they represent a cross-section of the
kinds of incident that can involve any
horse, at any type of yard. The signs are
often more subtle than symptoms of lameness, but they become quite obvious once
they are related to a definite situation.

There are two ways of establishing
whether or not the horse has a back
disorder: one is by feeling, the other is by
looking. The initial impression that something is not quite right in the horse's back
is often made during ridden exercise. The
rider can **feel** that the horse is not
responding to the commands in his accustomed manner, and the trainer may
observe changes in the horse's usual
stride. If a rider feels a resistance or difficulty that was not there before, this
should be taken as diagnostic.

There are a number of signs to look out
for:

• The horse does not want to move
straight down the long side of the arena;
for example, he moves his quarters in or
goes against the rider's leg.
• The horse is unbalanced at canter; he
is OK on one rein but cannot strike off on
the other, goes disunited or constantly
changes legs.
• The horse is unable to change diago-
nals fluently at the trot, from one large
circle to another.

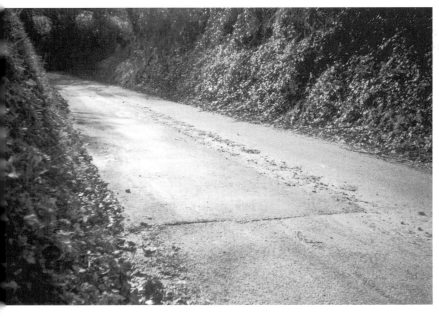

*Bad for
backs:
slippery
tarmac.*

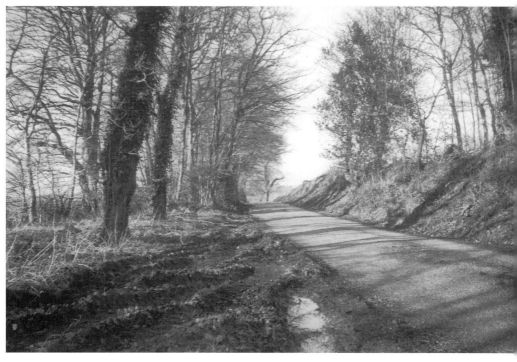

Bad for backs: an abrupt change of going.

• The horse goes wide behind when asked for lengthened strides at the trot.
• The horse has difficulty walking in a straight line down an incline.
• The horse appears to 'run out of steam' going up hill.
• Unlevelness in the fore- and hind-limb strides, at different times, and at different gaits.
• The horse is unable to bring the hind feet into the footsteps of the forefeet.
• The horse is unwilling to lower the head carriage, and accept the bit. This may affect only one gait, or even one level of collection in one gait, depending on the severity of the problem: for example in trot or, in particular, extended trot.
• The horse is unable to follow the tracks of the forefeet with the hind feet on a

circle. For example, the inner hind foot goes into the footstep of the outside fore foot, and the outside hind foot goes wide.
• Tension in the back behind the saddle; the rider feels he is sitting 'downhill'.
• Loss of contact with one side of the back under the rider's seatbone.
• The rider feels one stirrup is longer than the other when they are actually identical.
• The rider feels twisted in the saddle, or his jacket twists around him when the horse is trotting.
• The saddle keeps slipping to one side.
• The rider has a sore back after riding.

These should always be considered as possible indications of a back disorder, even though a thorough investigation

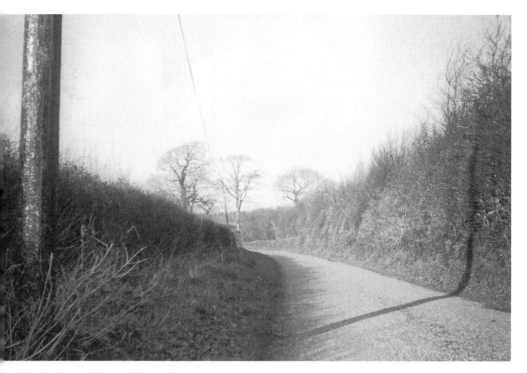

…ad for backs: endless walking along the camber of the road.

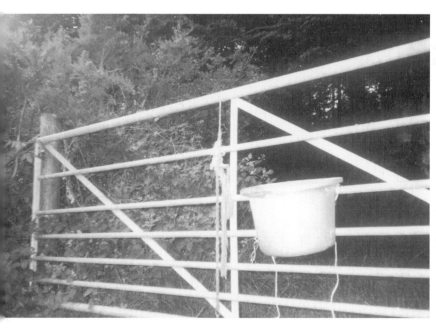

Bad for backs: pulling backwards while tied up, especially if the gate comes off its hinges.

61

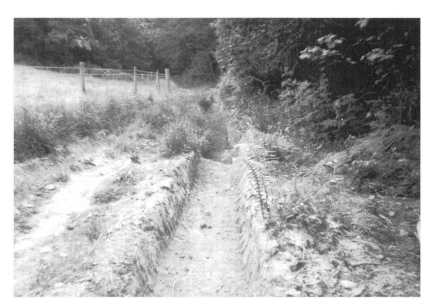

Bad for backs: stepping suddenly into a deep rut.

must be carried out to eliminate any other clinical conditions.

The next step is to **look** for discrepancies in the skeletal frame or muscle build. If the problem is very recent, the asymmetry may be only slight, but if the horse has been avoiding using a painful part of his back for any length of time there will be a marked difference in muscle development on each side of the horse.

Typical physical indications include the following:

• At the poll, there is uneven muscle development on the left and right sides of the Atlas bone. View from behind the horse.
• Enlarged muscles in front of the shoulder-blades, on one side only or on both sides. View from in front of the horse.
• Enlargement of the rear portion of the pectoral muscles, usually just behind where the girth would lie.
• Overbuilt muscles at the withers giving the horse a hunched-up appearance
• Loss of muscle behind the shoulder blades, under the points of the saddle-tree
• Loss of hair *anywhere* under the bearing surface of the saddle.
• Small raised plaques, often appearing in the saddle area.
• Hollows in the long back muscles, from the size of a ten pence coin to the area covered by the palm of the hand.
• Raised dorsal spinous processes possibly only one or two, in the mid-back or throughout the entire profile of the lumbar portion of the spine (roach back).
• Lumbar longissimus muscles that are raised higher than the tips of the dorsal spinous processes, on one side only or on both sides of the spine.
• A difference in the height of the bones of the sacro-iliac joint. View from behind the horse.
• A difference in the profile of the gluteal muscles and prominence of

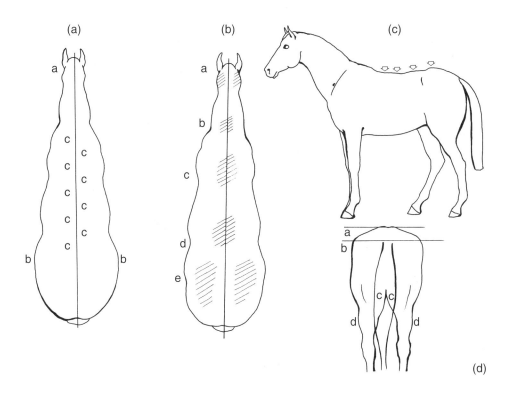

Visible points of musculoskeletal asymmetry.
(a) Bony landmarks: a, wings of the Atlas; b, points of the hips; c, dorsal spinous processes.
(b) Asymmetrical muscle development: a, at the poll; b, in the front of the withers; c, over and
behind the withers; d, over the loins; e, in the quarters.
(c) Irregularities in the heights of the dorsal spinous processes, and at the lumbosacral junction.
(d) Landmarks of asymmetry seen from behind the horse: a, the sacro-iliac joints (tuber sacrale);
b, points of the hips (tuber coxae); c, muscle development in the groin; d, muscle development in
the gaskins.

the points of the hips. View from behind the horse.
• Very pronounced development of the gaskins.
• Any variance of shape between the muscles on the insides of the hind limbs. View from behind the horse, lifting the tail to one side.

Any of the above are diagnostic of over- or underuse of muscles.

Such changes in muscle build may be caused by pain local to the area, or they may be a consequence of avoiding pain anywhere else along the back. Whether they are primary indications or secondary symptoms of compensation, they are going to need rebalancing.

An important element in the diagnosis of back disorders is the ability to feel what is going on below the skin's surface, and then to visualize, in your

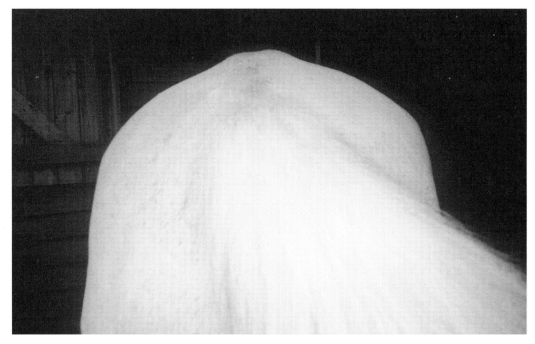

Severe skeletal asymmetry in an aged Thoroughbred.

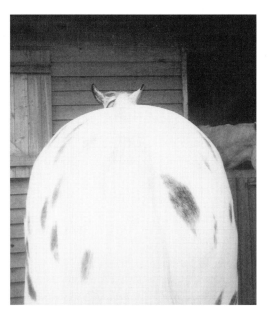

Marked asymmetry in the left and right gluteal muscles.

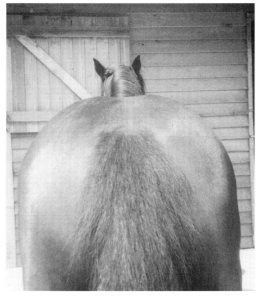

Slight asymmetry in the profile of the sacro-iliac joint.

mind's eye, how this may relate to any awkwardness of movement. Developing a diagnostic sense of touch is necessary for anybody training to treat back problems professionally – physiotherapists, chiropractors, even saddlers. Yet the layperson can gain a lot of information about his horse by practising palpation of the back, even though the actual interpretation may need professional assistance. After all, most people do not hesitate to feel down their horse's legs when they think there might be a lameness, and from this they are usually able to make some preliminary judgement. Palpation as an aid to diagnosis simply means being critical of what you can feel, in the same way that one is critical of the horse's response to the aids when riding. What you are feeling for is:

• Variations in temperature. This indicates a difference in blood circulation in that area: too hot would indicate inflammation, too cold would indicate reduced blood supply, or ischaemia.
• A difference in muscle tone beneath the skin. Increased muscle tone feels very hard to the touch, like a wooden board. Loss of muscle tone feels like cotton wool under the fingers, as though there is no real body substance under the skin.
• Heightened sensitivity, or loss of sensitivity. There are nerve-endings at approximately 2in (5cm) intervals all the way along the back. The horse should flex his back muscles slightly when these are activated. Intense twitching in any area of the back – sometimes before the hand has even made contact – should be regarded as an abnormal response. If part of a back muscle feels like a lump of heavy clay under the fingers (often a symptom in the lumbar region), there is almost

certainly loss of nerve transmission at this point.
• Pain.

If you touch a horse somewhere, and he kicks you, or makes a face, or threatens in any way, unless it is a particularly ticklish area most horse people would assume the horse is in pain. However, when it comes to back pain there are an awful lot of misconceptions, and therefore expressions of pain can go unheeded until the horse develops a severe behavioural problem, or loss of co-ordination. If you or I experience a shooting pain in the back, our typical reaction is to stand absolutely still, and (usually) to clutch at the bit that hurts. This signals to other people not to come anywhere near because we are especially vulnerable in such a condition. The body gives out very clear warnings in order to protect the integrity of the spinal cord.

What can the horse do? He can stand still, or he can run away. On the one hand he gets accused of napping, on the other he is described as bolting. If the incidents of pain recur, and he makes any response at all, he is labelled as difficult. There are horses that lay their ears back, roll their eyes and swish their tails whenever the rider walks into the stable carrying a saddle, and yet it never occurs to the person that the horse might be trying to express pain or, at least, the anticipation of pain, or that this might have anything to do with the horse's back!

THE LANGUAGE OF PAIN

When it comes to evaluating the presence of pain, there is no harm in being anthropomorphic: we should just try to imagine how *we* would feel. People who have had a horse for several years, and perhaps watched him grow older and a little less mobile, often confidently describe their horses as being a bit stiff in the mornings, but not in any pain: *how do they know?* Stiffness in muscles is a symptom of pain, as is stiffness in joints. The pain can be ignored, by horses as well as humans, and it can be overcome, but that doesn't mean to say it isn't there. If there hadn't been an element of pain, there would be no reason for stiffness in the first place.

When it comes to dealing with back disorders in the horse, it is very important to understand that there are different levels of intensity of pain. These different intensities are reflected in the way the horse attempts to communicate the sensation of pain to his human handler. Levels of pain are determined by the type of nerve or specialized receptor cell that transmits the signal, the density of these nerves in one area of tissue, and whether or not the signals reach the cerebral cortex and become conscious.

The sensation of pain falls into two broad categories: sharp pain and dull pain. However, if you think of any pain you have experienced, you will immediately realize that we humans use a variety of descriptions to communicate its exact quality: burning, throbbing, stabbing; or, it's like hot needles, it's like a ten-pound hammer, or a tight band around . . ., and so on. The horse can't verbalize his pain, but there is no reason to suppose that his pain does not have different qualities within the dull and sharp categories. The only way the horse can convey this is through his body language. Recognizing the language of pain in the horse is more important than knowing when your horse wants an apple or a carrot, especially if you're intending to sit on his back.

The horse's body language can be divided into three parts:

1. Changes in facial expression.
2. Changes in the posture of the whole body.
3. Changes in tail carriage.

He may use any combination of these three elements to express displeasure, discomfort or pain; and in addition he may express these things vocally.

Changes in Facial Expression

• Wrinkling one or both nostrils.
• Narrowing the eyelids.
• Showing the white of an eye.
• Rolling the eyes.
• Flattening one or both ears.

Changes in Posture

• Lifting the head and hollowing the neck and back.
• Flexing the back away from an approaching saddle or rug.
• Dipping the back when mounted (cold-backed).
• Threatening with flattened ears, hollowed back, and raised quarters, or lifting a hind leg.
• Excessive twitching when groomed.
• Fidgety when tied up.
• Hunching the back.

Changes in Tail Carriage

• Carrying the tail to one side.
• Clamping the tail to the hindquarters.
• Tail swishing.

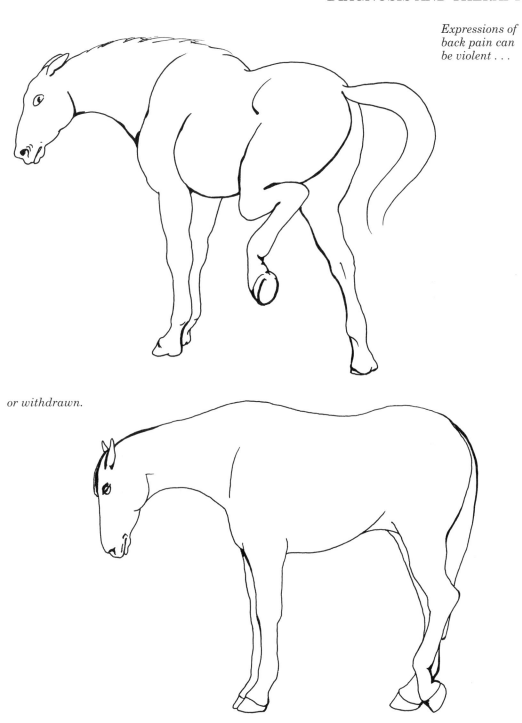

Expressions of back pain can be violent . . .

or withdrawn.

Vocal Expressions

- Grinding the teeth.
- Sharp intaking of breath.
- Grunting, for example, when ridden down an incline.
- Windsucking after, or even during, exercise.

The above list is not exhaustive, but it should give every horse person a clue as to the relevance of certain expressions in the horse's body language when deciding whether or not there is discomfort in the back. Having established in one's own mind that there is a problem to be investigated, it is time to call in professional assistance.

PROFESSIONAL DIAGNOSES AND THERAPIES

There is a competition coming up, possibly quite an important one, and the horse isn't going quite as well as expected. There's a bit of resistance here, a bit of unlevelness there, not quite going forwards enough, not quite coming through from behind. Who do you call? The back person. But what exactly *is* a back person, that he should be able to wave a magic wand over your horse's back and thereby restore those much-needed qualities of impulsion, 'throughness' and submissiveness in an instant? Back people are all around us, going from yard to yard, even treating horses between classes at the same competition, but what are their credentials and, more importantly, what do they really do?

Not so long ago, that would not have been such a difficult question to answer. A back person was a horseman, usually a good horseman, who understood how horses move and how blockages in that movement could be overcome by applying the principle of levers and no small amount of force. In addition they prescribed a period of rest along with some form of heat therapy. The horses got better for a time, but it was not unusual for the back person to have to repeat the treatment at regular intervals. Whether the successful resolution of a back problem was owed to the basic manipulation, the heat, or just the rest, we shall never know. However, it did give rise to a serious debate on whether horses' backs could, or should, be treated by manipulation, especially when practised by non-veterinarians.

At present, the effects of manipulation are still being disputed by the scientists. At the same time the credentials of the back people have changed enormously. There are now so many different ways of treating the horse's back that it is no longer the therapist that is in question, but rather the suitability of the therapy for the condition that has been diagnosed. *Diagnosis* – that is the crux of the matter. Many horses' backs are treated without a diagnosis, and many more with a diagnosis that is not properly understood. Of course, diagnoses often have to be the product of educated guesswork among any group of professionals. This is especially true in the case of the horse's back, which is too large to be penetrated by ordinary diagnostic imaging systems. Yet the current approach to treatment is, in many cases, not even based on informed deduction; it is more like choosing a therapy out of a mail-order catalogue! Sometimes, it will be what you really wanted, and sometimes it won't be anything like you thought it would be. Similarly, when a therapy chosen virtually at random doesn't work, people are desperately disappointed. If back disorders are approached with logic, all the therapies should be the right fit, and the outcome of treatment much more rewarding.

The treatment of back disorders falls into three categories:

1. An orthodox medical approach, which may include surgery.
2. The use of complementary medicines.
3. The support of the ancillary services to maintain a healthy framework for the back to work in: shoeing, saddlery, dental care, and training.

THE ORTHODOX MEDICAL APPROACH

It has to be said that the average horse person who suspects his horse has a back disorder does not automatically think of calling out the vet. Veterinarians have come in for a great deal of criticism where horse's backs are concerned because many vets that treat horses don't actually ride, or they ride only occasionally. Traditionally, the treatment of horses came after the treatment of cattle, sheep and pigs, which were economically more important. In a rural veterinary practice the person most likely to take care of the horse work was the one who was perhaps seen once or twice a week on the hunting field. Specialization in equine medicine has come about only quite recently as a result of the enormous increase in horse-riding as a popular sport. However, modern veterinary medicine has also become highly scientific, and there are definitely communication problems when

a horse owner calls in the vet to diagnose what the owner can only describe as a feeling! In one case the rider had simply been marked down in one movement of a dressage test because the horse went across the diagonal of the arena at extended trot with a few wide strides behind. Yet the rider wanted to know why. It is a bit like asking the police to get a conviction on the basis of circumstantial evidence; a movement defect that lasts for not more than half a dozen strides is flimsy evidence indeed when it comes to making a scientific judgement. However, the horse was found to have overriding dorsal spinous processes, and the problem was successfully resolved by surgery. Veterinarians think in terms of body tissue, bones, muscles and ligaments, rather than in terms of riding, such as impulsion and collection. However, when deciding on a suitable therapy, the former is actually of greater use than trying to treat a riding problem symptomatically and then, in frustration, reaching for the draw-reins, anyway!

In most countries, the veterinary profession is the only one legally entrusted with the care of animals, including horses. A thorough examination by a veterinary surgeon should be the first step in any investigation of a back disorder. There are undoubtedly injuries that respond quickly to the use of complementary therapies like physiotherapy, chiropractic or osteopathy. The experienced horse person may feel confident that this is the best way to relieve the horse's symptoms. That's fine, but make sure the vet knows too! Ask the vet if there is anything in the horse's previous medical history which might be a possible contra-indication for the use of, say, chiropractic. Explain the nature of the incident you think has caused the symptoms, and why you are thinking of calling in a physiotherapist, for example. There is always a small possibility that the horse's condition will worsen after treatment. It can happen. There may be an underlying condition that will affect the horse in a way that nobody could have foreseen. In such an event, veterinary help is certain to be needed. The vet will be in a much better position to assist if he already has some idea of the problem.

Whether you have a Grade A showjumper, a potential Derby winner or a retired children's pony, the veterinary examination of the horse's back should provide answers to the following questions:

1. Is the nature of the back disorder painful, mechanical, or perhaps both?
2. Is disease – such as a *Herpes* virus infection or azoturia – involved?
3. Is it a primary back disorder, or the result of compensation for problems elsewhere – in the feet, for example?

When the horse is examined at home in his own stable, there are two diagnostic procedures: observation and palpation. The horse should be looked at in the box for evidence of musculoskeletal asymmetry, as well as signs of local swellings or hair loss. The limbs and feet should be checked for symptoms of lameness. Foot balance and suitability of the shoes should be inspected. Later the horse should be observed moving on hard and soft surfaces, and lunged or ridden as necessary. All the saddles that might be used on the horse should be to hand, and the horse's teeth should be checked at the same time.

Palpation of the horse's back includes evaluation of the spinal reflexes. As discussed earlier, there are branches of nerves located approximately every 2in (5cm) along the back. These are dorsal branches of the spinal nerves: they leave the main nerve-stem and extend back into the muscles that lie parallel to the spine. The only visible muscles are the longissimus and iliocostalis muscles along the back, and the trapezius and latissimus dorsi muscles over the withers: the nerve response to palpation has to be taken as diagnostic for the underlying muscles as well. When you press on a nerve-ending, it produces a small reaction in that part of the muscle. This is the basis for testing back reflexes. The response should be equal all the way along the back without exception.

Ventral branches of the spinal nerves lie between the ribs. These can be stimulated by finger pressure in order to examine the horse's ability to arch his back. A point just behind the position of the girth, on the mid-line of the horse's breastbone, can be used to get the same effect. Finger pressure drawn down a line over the gluteal muscles will cause the horse to flex the muscles either side of the lumbar spine. The suppleness of the lower back can also be evaluated by pulling the dock of the tail, two or three times in succession, and watching the response of the muscles either side of the sacrum.

Evaluating back reflexes can be quite subjective. Some horses respond to the touch of a finger, some need a ball-point pen to bring their backs to life, and others don't respond to anything less than the stimulus of blunt-ended spurs! The important thing is that the response should be consistent for the individual horse. A sensitive animal should not have an area of his back which requires a hoof-pick to get a reaction, and the less sensitive animal should not suddenly start to flinch before the finger has even touched the skin. Stimulation of the back reflexes is sometimes met with surprise by the horse, especially if he is not particularly required to use his back when being ridden. However, if the reaction is one of resentment, or anger, this is definitely diagnostic.

No response at all means loss of motor transmission, and therefore local paralysis of the muscles. Such areas have often ceased to be painful but have caused serious mechanical problems elsewhere. Look out for painful areas of compensation.

Having demonstrated the presence or absence of pain, eliminated the possibility of disease, and established that the primary disorder *is* in the back (and not in the feet, the limbs or the brain), there are now three likely courses of action:

1. Prescribe short-term pain relief in the form of chemical medication.
2. Carry out more detailed investigation, using specialized diagnostic equipment.
3. Refer the horse for treatment by a complementary therapist in, for example, physiotherapy or manipulation.

Orthodox Medication

The types of medication most likely to be used in treating the horse's back are anti-inflammatory substances, possibly antibiotics, and some topical preparations, which may include a corticosteroid and perhaps an antifungal substance.

Skin irritations, especially those in the saddle area, can cause the horse considerable discomfort, so much so that the horse may develop the habit of hollowing away from the saddle, and resist all the aids to lift his back when ridden. There are important consequences for the back muscles and the vertebrae if this type of resistance carries on for too long. The most common skin problems are caused by insect bites or small accumulations of dirt and sweat, both of which lead to the formation either of painful lumps, or hard painless nodules which nevertheless cause pain through pressure on the tissues beneath the skin. Treatment requires meticulous hygiene, and the daily use of medicated washes and anti-inflammatory creams. Fungal infections cause the hair shafts to break, and this leaves the skin more susceptible to damage by rubbing. For this, treatment may include a course of internal medication if the fungal infection is spread over the whole body.

It should not be forgotten that the skin is a two-way system. It doesn't only have to withstand environmental attacks from outside, it is often under pressure from metabolic processes within the body. The skin is sometimes used as the great dumping ground for toxins and unwanted substances which the body cannot eliminate by any other means. The most obvious example is an allergic reaction to something the horse has eaten, manifesting itself as areas of oedema on the body's surface. However, the skin and hair are also very accurate indicators of nutritional balance and internal health, and the most appropriate medication may, in fact, be a suitable vitamin and trace-element supplement to rebalance the body's metabolism from within. Antibiotics will be prescribed wherever there is evidence of bacterial infection, and the choice of antibiotic will depend on the susceptibility of the germ involved. Humans experience tired and painful muscles when they have symptoms of flu, and there are certainly viral infections that have a similar effect on horses. Antibiotics do not eliminate viruses, but they do keep opportunist germs at bay, leaving the body free to deal with the virus itself.

The form of medication most commonly prescribed for the back disorder is the anti-inflammatory powder. There are several different types, all belonging to the 'non-steroidal anti-inflammatory drug' group of substances, to which human drugs like aspirin and paracetamol also belong. These chemicals affect the different chain reactions which cause inflammation, so that some conditions may respond to Phenylbutazone, while others may respond more to a substance like Flunixin.

Many horse owners are concerned and critical about the use of anti-inflammatory drugs in their horses because these drugs have acquired the reputation of only masking the symptom of pain rather than curing its cause. However, whilst pain is a normal physiological response to damage in the body, its presence can be counter-productive especially when it comes to managing back disorders. Pain makes muscles tighten and this causes a reduction in blood supply. Without good circulation, there is no means by which the products of damaged tissue can be transported away, or fresh blood can be supplied to encourage healing. Pain is caused by chemicals from the damaged tissues in the first place, and the situation simply becomes self-perpetuating. Relieve the pain, reduce the inflammation, and

you go a long way to restoring the circulation and initiating the healing process.

There are three situations in which anti-inflammatory medication is not only advisable but also desirable:

1. For the short-term management of acute, severe pain – as might be occasioned by, for example, strain of the lumbosacral junction, or the sacro-iliac joint.

2. For the control of pain and tissue reaction after surgery – after resection of the dorsal spinous processes, for example.

3. For occasional use, at a low-dose rate, in the control of pain in chronic conditions, and in conjunction with a complementary therapy – a typical example might be arthritis in older horses.

Back disorders in horses are complex affairs because they are influenced by so many additional factors, such as the saddle, the rider, and the balance of the feet. After the initial veterinary examination, it may be possible to form only a tentative diagnosis. It may be necessary to wait and see how the horse responds to a short course of medication. For this reason, the horse person often thinks he will be better served by going straight to a back therapist – he is more likely to get a definitive diagnosis. This is quite possible, but it will *only* be a diagnosis about the back, not about the rest of the horse. For example, if you take your car to a tyre centre, you can expect a lot of information about tyres, the same applies for gear-boxes and exhausts. However, if the engine is faulty, you will probably take the car to a garage for a general mechanical check-up. When it comes to investigating back disorders in the horse, think of your veterinary surgeon as the all-round mechanic; and save the specialists for after the preliminary examination.

At some point in the investigation it may become clear that additional information is needed: the response to medication or one of the complementary therapies might be mediocre, or the horse may continue to have a recurrence of symptoms. Further diagnostic techniques include:

- Blood-testing.
- Radiography.
- Scintigraphy.
- Ultrasonography.

Blood Tests

There are routinely two parts to a blood-test: the first establishes the level of red and white blood cells; the second provides information about chemicals associated with the internal organs and skeletal muscles. The blood cells and some chemicals give an indication of the general health of the horse – whether he may be anaemic, or coping with infection; muscle enzyme levels reflect the stability of the muscle-fibre membranes. Enzymes control biochemical reactions within cells, and although a small amount of them circulate in the bloodstream normally, it's only when the muscle wall becomes damaged that their levels rise significantly. The detection of muscle enzymes is used to diagnose and monitor recovery in cases of azoturia. However, it is possible to get a temporary rise in enzyme levels with *any* muscle damage, for example acute spasm, which may have nothing to do with the tying-up syndrome. The correct interpretation of blood results always depends on assessing more than one sample, taken at regular intervals, possibly over several weeks.

Radiography

Radiography (or X-rays) is a means of making bone structures visible. If you have ever had to have your horse's feet X-rayed you will know that the machine is placed not more than a few feet from the horse, and that the plates are held very close to the hooves. Because of the roundness of the horse's body, getting clear pictures of the horse's spine requires a more powerful machine than can be transported to your own stable. It is possible to get views of the tops of the spinous processes at the withers using a transportable machine, but that is about all. Radiography of the horse's spine therefore means taking the horse to a specialist equine clinic. The horse is usually referred to a clinic for detailed investigation, so it is likely that the neck, and possibly even the head, will be X-rayed too. It is possible to X-ray the pelvis but this requires the horse to have a general anaesthetic as he has to be turned upside down.

Pictures of the back are taken as an overlapping series, often with the use of markers, so that the exact location of any lesions can be identified. Radiographs of the back provide information about:

- The relative positions of the dorsal spinous processes – whether they are inflamed by being too close together, or even overriding completely.
- The presence of fractures.
- The development of spurs of bone or arthritis which might cause damage to the spinal nerves.

Nuclear Scintigraphy

This method of investigation involves injecting a radioactive marker substance into the bloodstream, and then monitoring the way it is taken up by both bones and soft tissue throughout the whole body. Bone can be remodelled by the body not only after a fracture, but as a response to inflammation or mechanical overload. The marker substance accumulates wherever this remodelling is taking place, and by passing a detector over the body so-called hot spots can be located. The exact nature of the bony changes can then be made visible using X-ray pictures. Soft-tissue injuries can also be detected by this means, and then subsequently investigated by the appropriate method – in the case of a muscle, by diagnostic faradism; in the case of the supraspinous ligament, by ultrasonography. Scintigraphy is an excellent way of looking into the whole musculoskeletal system at one go, and it is especially useful when trying to decide whether the symptoms of a back disorder are owed to a primary cause in the back, or are a secondary consequence of compensation for pain elsewhere, such as arthritis in the hocks or developmental problems in the stifle. However, the results of scintigraphy are open to interpretation, and it is important that all the evidence is collected before the symptoms are evaluated.

Ultrasonography
Ultrasound scans are routinely used in the diagnosis of pregnancy. They are also used to detect lesions in the tendons and suspensory apparatus of the horse's limbs. More recently, diagnostic ultrasound has been used to locate areas of damage in the nuchal and supraspinous ligaments, structures which have a consistency very similar to that of the horse's tendons. Ultrasound used for medical purposes works on the same principles as that used by bats and submarines to find their way

about: by measuring the echo of ultrasound waves which bounce off surfaces around them. Diagnostic ultrasound waves are absorbed and reflected differently by the various kinds of tissue. Separation of ligament fibres and areas of haemorrhage can be deduced from any lack of uniformity in the reflected ultrasound beam.

From Diagnosis to Surgery

The wider availability of high-powered X-ray machines has meant that the investigation of back disorders in the horse can now be carried out on much the same lines as any routine lameness investigation. It is even possible to use local anaesthesia in the back because X-rays can be used to check the position of the needles. In the same way that nerve-blocks or intra-articular blocks are used to locate the site of pain in a limb, small amounts of local anaesthetic are injected between the dorsal spinous processes. Pain here can be temporarily relieved to the extent that a horse is able to move completely normally, even when ridden. When a back disorder has existed for a considerable length of time, and the horse has built up a number of compensatory movements, the ability to categorically locate the prime site of pain in this way is diagnostically and economically very important.

The orthodox approach to diagnosing back disorders therefore consists of:

Observation Musculoskeletal asymmetry and stride deviations.
Palpation Muscle function, nerve function (reflexes), and pain.
Regional anaesthesia Pain elimination.

Imaging

Radiography and nuclear scintigraphy: bone damage, new bone formation, cartilage and soft tissue lesions.

Thermal imaging: means of detecting reduced blood supply and therefore loss of muscle function, using infra-red light.

Ultrasonography.

Diagnostic faradism Muscle function and strength.

Blood-testing Disease and muscle metabolism.

The only structures that are hard to examine by any direct means are the many small ligaments that criss-cross the spine between each of the vertebrae. Although the tops of the dorsal spinous processes can be X-rayed, the bodies of the vertebrae are hidden deep beneath muscles and in the thorax, underneath the heads of the ribs. Misalignment of the vertebral bodies – caused by a ligament overstretching or tearing – is hard to demonstrate because X-rays are only two-dimensional pictures. Ligaments themselves do not show up on X-ray photographs. A diagnosis of ligament damage, therefore, has to be made after all the other evidence has been collected; it is really arrived at by a process of elimination.

It is now possible to diagnose accurately the physical cause of back disorders in the horse, just as it is in humans. However, just as in human medicine, the choice of therapy within the orthodox field is limited, the most important contribution being made by corrective surgery. In the case of the horse this is mainly restricted to resection of small areas of bone between the dorsal spinous processes when these have become so close as to bang into one another or even overlap. This operation has a good success rate provided no compromises are made during the period of convalescence. However, it has to be said that the post-operative rehabilitation of the horse usually falls to the owner, with only short-term, specific advice from the surgeon, whose involvement often ends once the stitches or staples have been removed (a period of about two weeks). It is often six months before the horse can be expected to return to ridden work, and many owners feel that this period of time should be used constructively to rebuild the back, to ensure that the same condition does not recur. In fact, this is a consideration for many people whose horses are laid off with a back disorder: what to do, where to go, who to ask? As in human medicine, the solution to many back disorders is to be found amongst those therapies that are collectively known as complementary medicine.

COMPLEMENTARY THERAPIES

Natural, holistic, herbal, alternative: these descriptions are applied to forms of medicine that are outside the orthodox approach. The words suggest that these therapies are somehow safer to use than orthodox medicines, either because they contain natural ingredients, or because they encourage the body's own natural healing resources. For this reason we might be tempted to think that they are relatively harmless if, for instance, we should accidentally choose the wrong one. In fact, most people would probably consider the consequences of being given an incorrect prescription by the doctor to be rather more serious than taking the wrong herbal medicine or being given the wrong homoeopathic remedy. Far from it! What we are dealing with in non-orthodox medicine, is a potent stimulus to the body's energy. It can be delivered by a number of different means, and it is capable of changing both the physical *and* the mental state of the patient.

The body runs on a mixture of chemistry and physics. The chemicals are contained in the air we breathe and the food we eat, which combine together to form the building blocks for the cells and, ultimately, all the different types of tissue, from muscles and nerves to a liver or a kidney. Every biological process is a chain of chemical reactions. However, these reactions require energy to get started, and they produce energy while they are taking place. Moreover, the body needs an information system to co-ordinate this chemical activity. This is carried out by nerve-cells, which transmit their information using electrical impulses. In fact, every cell in the body has its own electrical characteristics, and these create electrical gradients. The sum total of electrical activity, along with the energy produced by the chemical reactions, is best described as **bioenergy**. It is the science of physics, rather than chemistry, which deals with the interaction of energy and matter, and which can best predict the behaviour of bioenergy in the body.

Orthodox medicine is mainly concerned with chemical processes: when these begin to head off in the wrong direction, or get out of hand, orthodox medicine considers how they can be brought back into line by introducing other, usually synthetic, chemicals into the equation.

A completely different way of tackling a biological problem is to alter the body's physics. In other words, to manipulate the bioenergy, and change the chemistry as a consequence. Whether you call it holistic or alternative, this is the principle of all non-orthodox medicine.

In the case of treating backs, there are special considerations. The central structure of the back is the spine, and at the core of the spine are the nerves of the spinal cord. In terms of bioenergy this is a powerhouse. All the transmissions generated by the nerves in the body, as well as many of those made in the brain, pass along the spinal cord. The information buzzes back and forth, twenty-four hours a day, for an entire lifetime. Instructions are passed to and from the skin and the musculoskeletal system, and much of the activity of the internal organs is regulated via the spinal cord. The entire state of an individual's health is mapped out along his back, in horses just as in humans. Ancient civilizations recognized this, and developed not only medical treatments but philosophies of life using the back as a focal point. It is no exaggeration to say that the back reflects changes in the condition of the entire body's bioenergy, like a barometer measures changes in the weather.

Using any form of medicine that directly manipulates the body's energy should not be done lightheartedly. This kind of medicine is a great deal more potent than most of us would ever dream! For this reason it is advisable to have a means of double-checking the results of treatment, and this is often best done by using the facilities offered by orthodox medicine. Of course, energy medicine in any form has its own system of diagnosis and doesn't depend on the confirmation of X-rays or nuclear scintigraphy to be successful. Nevertheless, when this kind of information *is* available, it may be used to indicate the most appropriate non-orthodox treatment.

Every type of energy medicine has its strengths and weaknesses and it is often beneficial to use therapies in combination. For this reason it is almost preferable to refer to them as complementary therapies, rather than alternative, because the objective is to pool the resources of both the orthodox *and* the non-orthodox, of the chemistry *and* the physics.

Medicine that uses the body's physical as opposed to chemical properties originated hundreds if not thousands of years ago. However, that is not to say that there was no form of chemical healing. The ancient Chinese, Indian, American and Australasian civilizations all had plants and herbs which were valued for their medicinal qualities. The pharmacologically active ingredients of plants were used to complement the effects of stimulating the body's energy field. Even today, the practitioner of traditional Chinese medicine, for example, is not just somebody who practises acupuncture: he is also a herbalist, and his treatment will require both these skills. For this reason, we should not feel obliged to be 'purists' when it comes to using energy medicine. Even if, today, our choice of chemicals is of the synthetic variety, the use of chemicals is an age-old medical tradition – combined, as they were, with other forms of healing; and there is no reason why we should not do the same.

Many of the complementary therapies available today have been developed relatively recently. They were created by great observers and original thinkers who had become disillusioned with the blinkered views of the medicine of their time, like Dr Samuel Hahnemann, the father of homoeopathy, Dr Edward Bach, originator of the Bach flower remedies, and Dr Andrew Still, the founder of osteopathy.

What all these men had in common was that they focused not on the disease but on the individual patient. (We have only to think of our own modern pharmacy, where drugs are prescribed to suit the illness, not the patient, to appreciate how their approach differed from that of their contemporaries). This meant that in assessing a patient's condition they took into account the person's emotional and physical make-up as well as the presenting symptoms of their illness. For example, two people suffering from influenza may exhibit very different symptoms and, what is more important, have entirely different states of mind. The one may have a fever and a cough, the other may have a headache and muscle pains; the one may have to go to bed for a week, the other may carry on in spite of feeling unwell. It is the same virus that causes the illness, but the patient's response is quite individual. When the illness is treated by addressing the body's energy level, the therapy is matched to the individual need; the one patient requiring a lot of support, the other perhaps only a 'nudge'.

To manipulate bioenergy therapeutically, you have to use instruments which either conduct electricity or produce electromagnetic waves, or which are capable of introducing energy patterns into the body. This is really nothing less than a description of physiotherapy machines – faradic stimulation, laser light, or ultrasound. In fact, physiotherapy is a modern form of energy medicine. However the very 'simplest' instrument for manipulating bioenergy is the human hand. It is also possibly the most versatile. It can change the alignment of bones, and release energy blocks; it can act as a conductor, allowing stored and unwanted energy to 'earth'; or it can help healing energy to circulate more positively round the body. Manipulation of the spine takes place at many levels; it's not just thrusts and cuffs that can change the position of the vertebrae. So much of the body's bioenergy is concentrated along the spine that, with heightened awareness, the touch of a single finger can produce profound changes in the body, using the spine as a medium.

Modern orthodox medicine does use selective forms of bioenergy for diagnosis: it measures the electrical impulses to the heart (electrocardiography), to the brain (electroencephalography), and muscles (electromyography). However, the use of electricity as a therapeutic stimulus has remained either crude, as in the shock therapy for the treatment of mental illness, or extreme, as in the application of the defibrillator in emergency stimulation of the heart. The body's bioelectricity is measured in millivolts: it might make your skin tingle, your heart beat faster, or your ears hum a bit, but it certainly isn't meant to make your hair stand on end, or fry you to a crisp. Compared to the electrical energy measured during medical diagnosis, the energy in the body as a whole is as different as images seen through a magnifying glass are different to those seen through a microscope. Orthodox medicine has not yet translated diagnostic energy into therapy; it still prefers to work with chemical compounds. These may modify the body's energy patterns, but they don't necessarily correct and heal them.

The back carries such a substantial amount of the flow of bioenergy that it lends itself not only to treatment of its own disorders by energy medicine, but to the treatment of disorders affecting limbs and organs. By its very nature, treatment of the back is treatment of the whole body. It is holistic. Moreover, medicine that uses the body's energy cannot make a distinction between physical and mental symptoms because the energy is produced during both physical and mental activity. There are no boundaries.

Back disorders bring with them a variety of emotions, both in humans and in horses: anxiety, restlessness, depression, anger. A physical cure is seldom enough. For example, a horse is emotionally geared to moving forwards because it is an animal of flight, but a horse that is *made* to go forwards in spite of physical pain, especially in the back area, suffers mental distress and emotional conflict. This often remains after the physical problem has been solved. Horses carry the confidence of their personalities in their backs, and complementary medicines, which work via the body's bioenergy system, can play an important part in restoring this confidence.

Complementary therapies for backs include:

- Physiotherapy.
- Manipulation and touch therapies.
- Acupuncture.
- Homoeopathy and healing.

Practitioners of the individual therapies have their appropriate diagnostic tests. The physiotherapist may look at the range of movement in the back, the chiropractor may look at the alignment of the bones, the acupuncturist may test the response to reflexes, and the homoeopath may ask for behavioural symptoms. Each therapy is a self-contained system, and it is perfectly possible to achieve a cure using one therapy only. However, there is no harm – and usually every benefit – in

Warning

It sometimes seems convenient to forget that those who practise complementary medicine actually have professional training. In the individual disciplines, this training may take several years to complete and require years of practical experience to achieve proficiency. Whereas most people would not consider themselves sufficiently medically trained to prescribe an exact type of antibiotic, even though they are capable of giving an injection, there are people who think that all you have to know about an ultrasound machine, for example, is how to switch it on! There are even more unscrupulous people who claim to practise forms of manipulation – and take good money for doing so – even though they have no training at all. Needless to say, a great deal of harm is done, and not just to the horse owner's wallet. There are only two ways to safeguard yourself against being 'taken for a ride', and that is to check professional credentials and to find out something about the therapies themselves, before you hire the therapist.

is usually produced by machines, and it can therefore be given at a standardized dose rate. It is possible to prescribe a specific dose of electromagnetic energy or heat, for example, in a way that is not possible with other complementary therapies. The aim of physiotherapy is to speed up the healing process in tissue that is damaged; it does this by increasing the blood circulation and promoting the drainage of waste materials. This can be done manually, for example by massage, or by machines using ultrasound waves, electromagnetism, laser light, or the electrical stimulation of muscle/nerve complexes. Cells in damaged tissue change their electrical properties. Application of energy using a variety of physiotherapy machines stimulates the cells to return to their normal electrical patterns. This is the essence of healing.

Diagnostically, physiotherapy is closer to orthodox medicine than most other complementary therapies because it deals with specific tissue types, muscles, bones, nerves, rather than with diagnosing energy levels as such. The energy input is quantifiable; it is determined by the type of tissue to be treated. For example, ultrasound waves at too high a dose can burn. Other complementary therapies do not allow the same control over energy input or uptake, but for this reason can spread their energy more widely; the dangers of a local phenomenon, like a thermal effect, do not have to be considered.

Physiotherapy is concerned with mobilization, that is restoring movement to parts of the body that have become locked in spasm, or weak through inactivity. Such areas block or reduce the flow of bioenergy. Even though treatment by

cross-referencing, and in using two or more therapies either concurrently or in quick succession. The art of using complementary therapies is to pool the results of both the successes *and* the failures, to achieve a truly holistic form of medicine.

Physiotherapy

Physiotherapy is the most modern form of energy medicine. The therapeutic energy

79

physiotherapy tends to focus on a specific area of disability, the removal of one obstacle – for example spasm in the lumbar muscles, or imbalance in the sacro-iliac joint – can restore the flow of bioenergy. A physiotherapist should be consulted when the back disorder involves:

• Muscle spasm.
• Loss of muscle tone or substance.
• Loss of nerve transmission.
• Lesions in the supraspinous ligament.
• Damage to soft tissue, such as ligaments and fascia.
• Pain.

Under instruction from a qualified physiotherapist the following treatments may be appropriate for backs:

Local ice-packs To reduce swellings and encourage circulation.
Heat treatment With infra-red lamps, for example, to create deep heat and relax muscles.
Ultrasound To reduce swellings and promote healing (but to be used very cautiously anywhere near the spine).
H-wave The use of combined electrical currents to increase the circulation and relieve pain. Used to speed healing in deep-seated soft-tissue injuries in the horse's back, but best left to the professionals.
Laser light 'Cold' or low-powered lasers are used to encourage healing. They are especially beneficial near nerves.
Magnetic therapy For pain relief, promoting circulation, and relaxing muscles.
Trophic muscle stimulation Produces muscle contraction by sending an impulse to the nerve. It is more physiological than faradism, which can be painful

when used on muscles that are already sore, and it is a good way to rebuild specific groups of muscles when these have wasted through injury. It is usually carried out by the owner; treatment is daily over several weeks.

Most physiotherapy treatment stimulates the release of endorphins in the patient. Endorphins are a group of chemicals that are produced by the body to relieve pain. Their release is a feature of all complementary therapies, and it seems to invoke deep relaxation and even a mildly euphoric state in horses undergoing treatment.

Manipulation and Touch Therapies

Of all the treatments that are used on backs, manipulation is the most controversial, at least where horses are concerned. The majority of horse owners call in the back person (that is, the manipulative therapist) whenever they think their horse has a back disorder, yet the majority of vets remain sceptical or dismissive about the benefits of such a treatment.

A major stumbling block to the veterinary profession's acceptance of manipulation as a valid form of treatment, is the use of the word 'out' as a diagnostic term. The concept of 'outness' lacks scientific precision, and although it is understood by most horse people – in the same way that through (the back) or over (the back) are understood in the vocabulary of riding – many equine veterinary surgeons are reluctant to use this popular expression because it is so open to misinterpretation. Most of the veterinary profession also strongly contests the idea that the vertebrae of a horse's back can be moved by the strength of the average human being, using only his hands. There is some concession towards manipulation of the bones in the horse's neck, but there is scepticism about adjusting the position of the rest of the horse's spine because of the way it is encased by sizeable muscles and other soft tissue. Nevertheless, the horse world as a whole continues to employ back manipulators, and presumably would not do so if there were not obvious improvements in the horses after treatment, whatever the doubters in the veterinary profession might say. What, therefore, can be achieved by having a horse's back manipulated? How is it done, and how does it work?

The precise alignment of the vertebrae is of great importance to the body, because these bones protect the nerves of the spinal cord. Any deviation in this long, segmented, bony tunnel pinches the nerve-fibres and stops them transmitting information. Nerves exit the tunnel at every junction between the vertebrae and these, too, are in danger of being squashed or even severed, if the relative positions of the vertebrae change. There is a complex feedback system at the intersections of the vertebrae to ensure that the exit holes maintain their specified dimensions. The vertebrae themselves are interlocked by small bony protrusions, but their overall positions are governed by the elastic strength of the ligaments and the tone of the surrounding muscles. In the event of trauma, caused by concussion, jarring, overstretching of ligaments and the like, it is the muscles that have to retain the alignment of the spine in order to protect the integrity of the spinal cord. This may mean that a portion of muscle contracts to

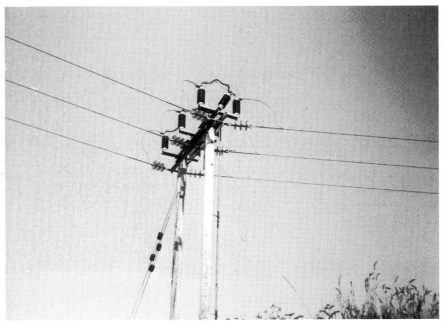

Nerves have a complex feedback system at every intervertebral junction.

its shortest length, effectively pulling that part of the bone to which it is attached, out of line with adjacent vertebrae. Muscle spasm is the body's way of protecting itself against further injury, but at the same time it sets up asymmetry along the spine. After a time, this begins to affect the balance of the limbs and more distant areas of the back and neck. Unfortunately, muscle spasm will remain, sometimes for several years, until it is actively released. The body simply works round it.

A common site for this type of restriction is around the pelvis. The pelvis supports the large gluteal muscles of the quarters. To the rider, these muscles are the engine of the horse, the place where impulsion and collection are generated. Not many people think of the pelvis as housing important internal organs, which have to be protected at all cost. Overstretching a back leg, for example over an awkward jump, down a slippery track, or even just on a smooth piece of tarmac, is not an uncommon occurrence for horses. However, the horse's body is more concerned with protecting the large intestine, the bladder and the reproductive organs, than its ability to do left and right circles with equal balance. The muscles of the quarters immediately go into spasm to protect the pelvic ring from being dislodged and causing damage to the vital organs. This causes considerable imbalance in the movement of the quarters.

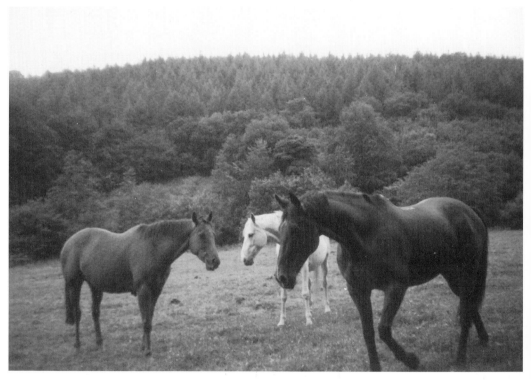

Good for backs: freedom of movement.

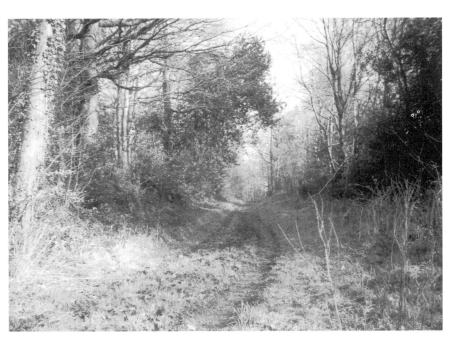

Good for backs: forward movement along an inviting track.

It gradually transfers itself along the back, affecting the tone of the muscles either side of the lumbar spine, throwing the saddle off centre, and eventually twisting the neck, as the horse tries to create an area of counterbalance at the poll. When horses experience difficulties with their flatwork on one particular rein, it is often because one part of the pelvis is significantly in front of, or lower than, the equivalent part on the opposite side. This condition will sometimes respond to treatment with anti-inflammatory powders if, at the same time, a specific exercise regime is carried out by a skilled trainer. However, the process is time-consuming and the end result never entirely satisfactory. Manipulation, on the other hand, is immediately effective; although, in long-standing disorders, it still does not eliminate the need for a programme of careful rehabilitation.

The diagnosis of outness does not refer to the whole vertebra: this would be equivalent to a dislocation. Instead, it refers to one part of the vertebra which is pulled at an angle, compared to the adjacent bones. So, to manipulate the back, it is not necessary to manhandle the entire skeleton! Imagine a row of fencing posts with a strand of wire running between them. It is easy to see at a glance when one post is tilted out of line, yet to bring it back into the upright position again it is not always necessary to take a hammer to the post. You could simply adjust the tension of the wire. By altering the tone of the muscles along the back (and neck, and pelvis) the angle of the vertebrae can be corrected. This relieves compression on the vital structures around and between the vertebral bodies.

Many people are familiar with the physical techniques of manipulation used by

83

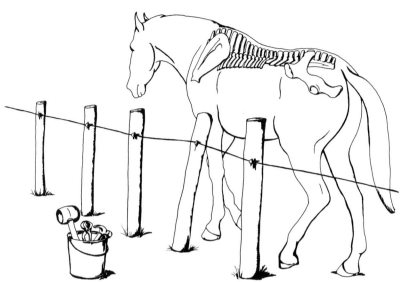

A fencing post can be pulled back into line using different mechanical forces. The same is true of the horse's spine.

chiropractors and osteopaths. These two schools of manipulation have different origins, but they share a common philosophy, that manipulation of the spine improves the health of internal organs by freeing the nerves which control their function. Both types of manipulation improve the flow of bioenergy along the spine and all round the body because they release the muscle spasm which causes this energy to be diverted or to stagnate. Once this flow is restored, there is an improvement in blood circulation and any traumatized tissue can be repaired.

The spine carries so much of the body's bioenergy that it is especially susceptible to therapeutic techniques, which are more subtle than physical manipulation. It is possible to change the tone of the muscles by altering the energy flow itself. In the example of the fence posts and wire, this would be the equivalent of changing the tension of the wire by applying some form of electronic tuning device, rather than using a mechanical tool. Such therapies combine massage with specialized touch techniques. They influence the electromagnetic energy flowing through the muscles which is produced by the nerves.

Horses are sensitive to the lightest form of touch, and many will respond with deep relaxation to a sympathetic hand laid quietly on the back. Light touch can create a healing environment in the horse's back, even when practised by an untrained hand, and it is particularly useful for restoring confidence in a horse that has experienced pain associated with the saddle. These horses often create their own misalignments along the spine when they are about to be tacked up, anticipating the pain of previous experience. They then find it difficult to work evenly through their backs during schooling, and are often severely 'one-sided'. Touch therapy is a means of providing reassurance as well as healing.

Many manipulation techniques are very immediate in their therapeutic effect, and there is a great temptation to use them as a 'quick fix', even just minutes before a competition. Both manipulation and massage may be justifiable to relieve jarring and prevent stiffening between strenuous events; they may even be a sensible precaution. However, when the musculoskeletal system becomes tired, it also becomes vulnerable. Manipulation can give the body a temporary reprieve, but it cannot instantaneously replace strength in tissues suffering from severe energy depletion. On the contrary, it is more likely to make them susceptible to serious injury. Furthermore, whenever an area of restricted movement has existed for any length of time, the underlying tissues will also have been out of action. When the restriction is released, these tissues will be weak and unaccustomed to prolonged periods of exercise. They need time to regain their strength and elasticity, to match the performance of other parts of the body which are already thoroughly trained. In this context, manipulation, as well as the more subtle touch therapies, should form part of an overall programme of physiotherapy.

Manipulation skills are now taken from many different sources, both ancient and modern. The back person is no longer somebody who has to use a great deal of physical effort to achieve a result. In fact, the less the actual physical force used, the deeper the therapy is likely to penetrate.

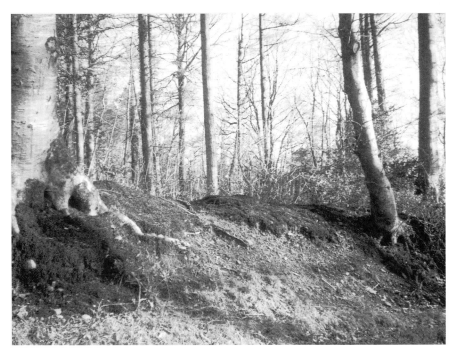

Good for backs: suppling the back by riding up and down small inclines.

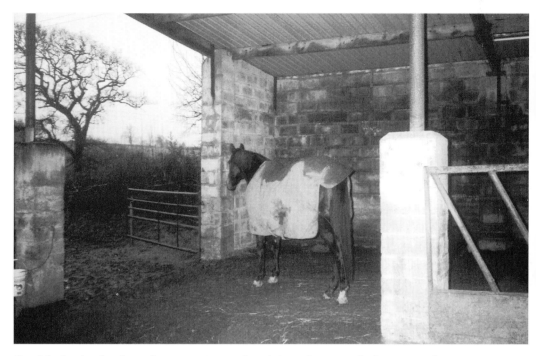

Good for backs: freedom of movement, even in winter – for example, in an open barn system.

It is potentially able to affect not only the physical alignment of the body but also its mental balance.

Therapies which might be considered for treatment of back disorders in the horse (ranging from those requiring some degree of physical force to those which stimulate the flow of bioenergy by light touch) are:

- Osteopathy.
- Chiropractic.
- Shiatsu.
- Chinese massage.
- Acupressure.
- Tellington-Jones Team work.
- Bowen technique.
- Healing.

There are several derivations within these therapeutic groups; individual schools of practice have developed the techniques in different directions. Not all therapists are automatically licensed to treat animals, however beneficial a therapy might be. Some therapies may be gentle in their application, but all have a profound effect on the body. Therefore, if nothing else, make sure they are carried out with both the knowledge *and* (it is hoped) the approval of your veterinary surgeon.

Acupuncture

Acupuncture is a system of medicine which originated in China more than two thousand years ago. What relevance could

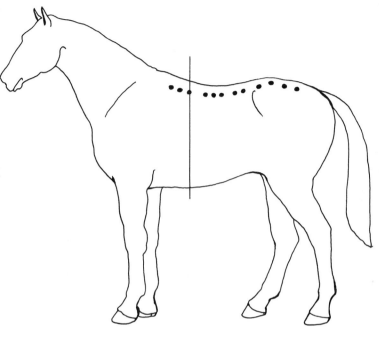

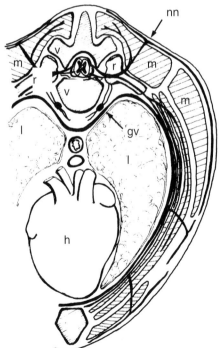

Acupuncture 'association' points along the horse's back correspond to meridians which are named after internal organs.
A cross-section through the horse at the position of the vertical line shows the vertebrae (v), ribs (r), muscles (m), sternum (st), heart (h), lungs (l), voluntary nerves (nn), and involuntary nerves (gv). The 'association' points are in close proximity to the voluntary nerves in the back muscles, but they also register changes in the involuntary nervous supply to the internal organs.

such a form of medicine have to sporting injuries in the modern horse? Could we even be put off exploring such a form of medicine because of its Oriental basis and possibly esoteric philosophy? As it happens, acupuncture is one of the most valuable and successful forms of treatment for back disorders in the horse, whether used on its own or as a complement to more orthodox treatments, such as surgery.

Acupuncture treatment is based on the idea that all the energy created by the biological processes in the body cannot stand still. The body's metabolism is dynamic and therefore causes the energy to move. As long as these metabolic processes are in balance, the energy flows in clearly defined channels, called meridians. However, when one element is affected by illness, the flow is changed; it may become weaker, or it may become a burden. Nevertheless the flow has to be re-established before health is restored. Imagine switching on all the electrical appliances in your home: the electricity will begin to flow through the wires. The wires are invisible because they are tucked away in conduits in the walls, but the amount of electricity can be measured, none the less. Switch one of the appliances off, and the strength of the electrical field will change. Acupuncture is based on a similar interpretation of the body's bioelectrical fields; these should be constant, when all the 'appliances' are switched on and working correctly.

The energy meridians are named after the major organs they pass through. Although there are said to be twelve individual meridians, they are really all joined in one continuous 'ribbon' that weaves its way in and out of the body. The

energy completes one entire circuit every twenty-four hours. The flow of energy is diagnosed manually by testing points along the meridians, where they are closest to the body's surface. The points lie either over blood vessels, especially in the limbs, or over nerves.

There is a series of important diagnostic points along the back, which can be used to confirm the presence of disorders anywhere in the body. The points lie over the superficial branches of nerves in the long back muscles. These link up to deeper branches of nerves close to the spinal cord. Through these connections, the back points can register either dysfunction in a vital organ in the corresponding segment of the body, or disorders along the external part of the meridian that bears that organ's name. The points are called association points. For example, there is an acupoint at the side of the withers, approximately at the place where the arch of the saddle tree rests on the horse. This is an association point for the lung. The lung meridian itself runs down the inside of the horse's forelimb. If the association point is tender or painful, this may indicate a forelimb lameness, an illness in the lung, or both. Other diagnostic points are then used to locate the problem precisely.

The association points along the horse's back are of relevance to the rider because he sits on several of them! If one or more of these points is sounding an alarm then the horse's back cannot be working comfortably. If the horse is not working fluently through his back, he must be compensating somewhere else, either in the neck, the quarters or the limbs. Areas of compensation develop tender points, and may even result in lameness. To an experienced acupunc-

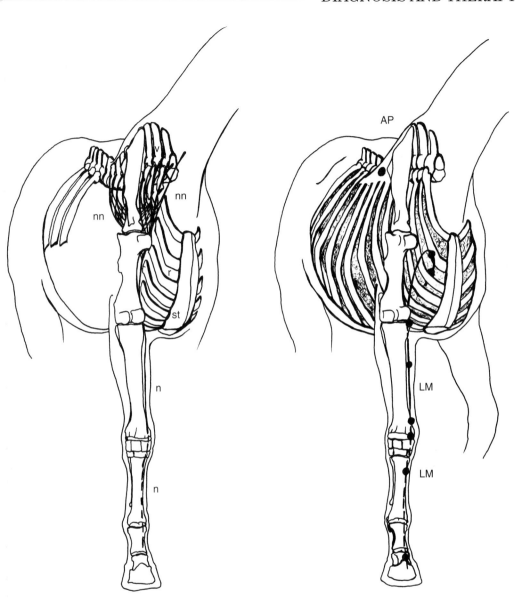

A single nerve, for example, the medial cutaneous nerve, which passes down the fore-limb of the horse, collects its component fibres from many different 'service tunnels' along the spine: st, sternum; r, ribs; v, vertebrae; nn, nerve-fibres; n, the cutaneous palmar nerve.

The course of the lung meridian (LM) follows the medial cutaneous nerve. Also shown is the position of the lung 'association' point at the withers.

turist, the location of these points and the presence of sensitivity in an association point of the back, can explain complex mechanisms of lameness, which do not yet receive the same kind of analysis in Western medicine. For example, a horse hollows away from the back of the saddle which is resting on the unsupported part of the lumbar muscles. A tenderness develops here at the association point of the stomach meridian. However, a horse that hollows in this way cannot lift his abdominal muscles and bring his hind

legs underneath his body, so he uses the base of the neck to keep his balance. The stomach meridian itself passes along the lower side of the neck, between the forelimbs, along the underside of the belly, through the stifle joint, and down the hind limb to the foot. A horse working with a flat or hollow back is likely to develop sore stifles. This can be confirmed by the presence of tender points along the course of the stomach meridian, coinciding with areas of musculoskeletal compensation. The principles of acupunc-

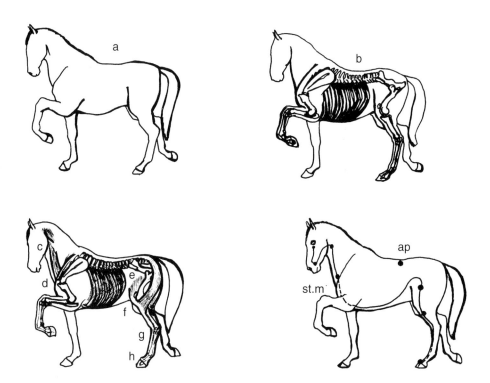

A training problem in the ridden horse translated into acupuncture diagnosis: a, the horse works with a hollow back; b, this creates discomfort at the thoracolumbar junction; the horse compensates, creating tension in the muscles marked c, d, e; and develops soreness in the stifle, hock and pastern joints (f, g, and h). The points of compensation are to be found along the stomach meridian, which has its 'association' point at the thoracolumbar junction.

ure have a great deal in common with the principles of riding!

Acupuncture treatment can be carried out in a number of ways. The most traditional method is to use needles, sometimes in conjunction with a herb called mugwort, which is left to smoulder close to the shaft of the needle. The acupoints are actually located below the skin's surface, so a more recent adaptation of the technique is to inject small deposits of a fluid, such as vitamin B12, using hypodermic needles. Traditional acupuncture needles are made of a single shaft of metal, which pushes its way through the tissue rather than cutting like a hollow needle. If the horse moves during treatment, there is sometimes a small amount of bruising, but this wears off very quickly. Acupoints can be stimulated by applying a small electrical current to the needles, or by the use of low-intensity laser light. The latter is particularly suited to treatment of the horse's lower limbs, although horses are not nearly as (acupuncture) needle-shy as one might imagine.

Acupuncture has several therapeutic effects. The first and most important, is to regulate the flow of bioenergy and redirect it along the correct channel if necessary. For example, when the needles are placed close to nerves, they have a significant influence on the electrical fields generated by those nerves. The effect is to release stored and unwanted energy from the surrounding tissue. Needling also stimulates the release of endorphins, the body's own pain-relieving substances, as well as increasing the levels of cortisol, which has anti-inflammatory properties, and serotonin, a substance which controls the constriction of blood vessels.

Horses receiving acupuncture treatment, often begin to make chewing movements with their jaws; they yawn and blink. They will lower their heads and go almost into a trance. This is presumably caused by the endorphin release, and it appears to be accompanied by deep relaxation. The sensation is obviously strange to the horse at first and some resist 'letting go' by latching onto sounds in their environment. For this reason acupuncture should be carried out in quiet surroundings, with the minimum of disturbance. The sensation of needling, however, is not unpleasant, as most horses relax very quickly and sometimes very dramatically at the second treatment. Horses that have previously been treated by chiropractic appear to have already experienced this sensation, and are often more immediately receptive to the effects of acupuncture needling.

Although the biological effects of acupuncture are now quite well researched and understood, nobody has yet been able to explain why the therapeutic effect should last in humans, sometimes for several years after even one treatment. In horses, four to six treatments are usually carried out on a weekly basis, but it is also possible to give the body gentle reminders at monthly or even yearly intervals. Acupuncture and manipulation combine well in the treatment of back disorders but, as with manipulation, the healing process initiated by acupuncture takes time. Essentially, we are asking the body to carry out its own repairs: it must be given time to do so.

Much of the body's bioenergy is accessible to the acupuncturist. Yet, even in traditional Chinese medicine, practitioners would not rely solely on this form of treatment. It would be combined with the introduction of an internal energy source in the form of herbal medicine. Chinese herbal medicine is not readily available to Western horse owners at present, so it has become more usual to combine acupuncture treatment with homoeopathy.

Herbs, Homoeopathy and Healing

When people talk of complementary medicine, they are inclined to use several 'H' words, as though they all mean the same thing: in particular, herbal, homoeopathic and holistic. Even though the horse world uses various forms of complementary medicine, there is just as much confusion as to the real meaning of these descriptions. Holistic, for example, means whole, and provided a therapy addresses the physical, mental *and* environmental imbalances which cause disease, it can justifiably be called holistic. Even orthodox medicine is holistic if it not only prescribes medication, but also takes into consideration the emotional symptoms and social pressures that might be contributing to the illness.

Therapies that stimulate the body's bioenergy system are more obviously considered to be holistic because the movement of energy is not bound by any anatomical restrictions. In fact, this energy is not even restricted by the body's shell: it interacts, and is affected by, the energies of the environment, which is why some types of illness can be related to the presence of high-tension electricity cables, nuclear-power stations, or excessive doses of background radiation. To be holistic, a therapy must look for imbalance in every quarter, not just in the physical symp-

toms. Herbalism and homoeopathy can be used holistically, but that doesn't mean to say they always are.

The holistic approach to the treatment of back disorders in the horse is likely to be made up of a number of different therapies and skills. For example, the saddler and the farrier will almost certainly be involved in the long-term management of a horse with a chronic sacro-iliac strain; they will form part of an holistic team. Herbs are available, both in feed and in supplements, and this too is a little misleading. Most horse people are, in effect, using a form of herbal medicine in their day to day feeding regimes, yet they cannot be said to be practising holistic medicine. Herbs contain substances which have medicinal qualities, and it is true that, with the advent of modern drugs, a great deal of the 'old' wisdom about the benefits of these plants has been ignored. However, the substances contained in herbs are still chemicals, even though they are not in injectable or powder form. The combination of naturally occurring ingredients is often more potent than the single synthetic counterparts, and herbs provide many more nuances of medicinal substances than are available in manufactured preparations. Nevertheless, the herbal mixtures currently available for horses are really a form of chemical medicine, even though this may provide some valuable nourishment for the body's bioenergy in a rather roundabout way.

Homoeopathy
Homoeopathy is quite different. Many of the ingredients used in homoeopathy are the same as in herbalism – hence the confusion – but while herbs have chemical

properties, homoeopathic remedies cannot be analysed chemically, and they are therefore probably better described as energy compounds. In fact, even though homoeopathy was invented a couple of hundred years ago, it may turn out to be a very advanced science altogether. In homoeopathy, a substance, which may be a plant, but might also be an insect poison, a snake venom or a mineral, is made into a solution. This solution is diluted many times over, to different strengths. It is not just the dilution which is important, but the fact that between the dilutions the mixture is shaken and tapped in a very specific way. This is by no means some quaint, archaic ritual. It is essential in ensuring that while the amount of the original substance becomes less in the stages of dilution, the therapeutic strength of solution actually becomes more powerful. This can only happen if something other than the molecules of the substance are being transferred and activated. It is thought that the shaking treatment of the solution between dilution stages (called succussion) transfers the imprint of an energy pattern which is specific to the original substances. In this way the energy is potentized at each stage.

The prescription of homoeopathic remedies is very different to that of orthodox medicines. Modern medicines are given because they oppose the symptoms of illness. Homoeopathic remedies are given because, in their natural, non-homoeopathic form, they would actually cause the symptoms that characterize the illness. For example, the symptoms of acute vomiting and diarrhoea could be caused by arsenic poisoning. Of course, they are usually caused by bacteria or a virus infection. Nevertheless, these same symptoms can be relieved by giving arsenic in homoeopathic dilution. When Dr Samuel Hahnemann carried out his first experiments, treating the symptoms of certain diseases by giving substances that would cause those symptoms in the healthy person, he was disappointed in the results. It was not until he decided to make the doses smaller (more dilute), rather than larger, that he started to achieve therapeutic success. Homoeopathic remedies are available in different potencies, as indicated by the number of times the remedy's substance has been diluted. A substance that has been diluted ten times will not be as potent as one that has been diluted 1,000 times. Therefore, contrary to what we are used to in orthodox medication, where 'more' means more effective, in homoeopathy 'more effective' definitely means less, that is, less of the working ingredient, but more of that ingredient's energy.

Once inside the body, a homoeopathic remedy behaves very differently to a chemical medicine. Chemical medicines slot into the same chemical process everywhere, as long as they are compatible with the tissue and can reach it via the bloodstream. A homoeopathic remedy slots into energy processes, anywhere in the body that is necessary, relieving groups of symptoms which may, at first, seem to have no common denominator. The two types of medicine can be compared to bank service-till cards: the card for orthodox medicine can be used at any branch of the same bank, but the card for homoeopathic medicine can be used at any branch of several affiliated banks as well. This gives homoeopathic medicine a wider therapeutic potential, which is especially valuable when treating back disorders.

Some homoeopathic remedies have a special affinity with certain types of tissue. For example, *Rhus toxicodendron* and *Ruta gravis* together cover most elements of the musculoskeletal system, and *Hypericum* has an affinity with nerve tissue. When the back is the focal point of treatment, stress to other parts of the body may go undiagnosed. When using homoeopathy, the whole body is automatically included in the treatment, even if some of the symptoms are secondary.

The transportation of homoeopathic remedies within the body is not apparently restricted to the bloodstream. They appear to be capable of interacting with energy processes anywhere, including the brain. Horses with back disorders experience a variety of emotional disturbances because the back is such a vulnerable part of their anatomy. Pain in the back affects one of the most deep-seated natural instincts in the horse: the fear of attack from a powerful predator. (No wonder some horses with back pain get angry, or violent!) Any treatment of back disorders in the horse should take into account the horse's emotional state. Orthodox medicine has recently taken to prescribing sedatives for humans with back pain. Yet while there are probably a lot of horses that would like to be on Valium, this solution has not yet found its way into equine medical practice! There are many homoeopathic remedies which include well-defined mental characteristics in their patterns of symptoms. These make a useful contribution to the treatment of horses that are emotionally out of balance because of back pain.

There are a number of remedies that are useful for musculoskeletal problems:

Arnica Any disturbance in blood circulation, from external bruising to internal shock.

Rhus tox Muscles and joint pain, when the symptoms are relieved by movement.

Bryonia Similar to *Rhus tox*, but preferred where the symptoms are aggravated by movement.

Ruta gravis Strain of tendons, ligaments, and pain in the periosteum.

Hypericum Damage to nerve-fibres.

Silica Skeletal weakness and general debility.

Berberis Pain in the lower back (lumbar muscles).

Herpes nosode Muscular debility and paralysis, caused by or similar to symptoms caused by this infection.

Some remedies have a strong mental component:

Aconitum Great fear or anxiety.

Argentum nitricum Apprehension.

Gelsemium Anticipatory fear, where the individual is quiet and subdued.

Ignatia Sadness; grief at losing a loved one.

Apart from *Arnica*, which is often used frequently (hourly or more) in a 6 or 30 potency, most of the other remedies will be more effective at 200 potency or above. Chronic conditions, namely those that have existed for more than three weeks, use up the energy of homoeopathic remedies very quickly, so that to begin with the treatment may have to be repeated every other day. However, there are some remedies that work well when given on an infrequent, occasional basis, but over a long period of time, like *Calc. fluor*, which has an affinity with bones.

There are many hundreds of remedies available in homoeopathy; in fact, anything can be made into a homoeopathic remedy, using the principle of dilution and succussion. Lists of remedies and their accompanying profiles of symptoms are published in books called *Materia Medica*. Not all the symptoms will be an exact match, because these details have been provided by the many people who were involved in 'proving' the remedies. It is necessary to sort out the most important symptoms, which give the closest match to those of the patient. It is rather like trying to unlock a door, and having perhaps twenty keys to choose from: one will be an exact fit, others may come close and some you can't even get into the lock. Therapeutic success is going to depend on how well the key turns the lock and opens the door.

Often, the most difficult part of any back therapy is restoring the mental balance and confidence of the patient. A horse that has experienced pain in his back gets scared. He may be very reluctant to risk moving in any way that might mean he is going to repeat the experience. It might make him defensive, aggressive or just fidgety. This behaviour can well outlast any physical problem. An extension of the homoeopathic principle, and one that is well worth considering in the long-term rehabilitation of horses with back disorders, are the Bach flower remedies. Dr Edward Bach who developed these remedies put the mental state of his patients before the physical, considering that physical symptoms could not respond adequately to treatment, if the patients were trapped in a negative frame of mind. By addressing the mental configuration of his patients he was able to give them relief from their physical symptoms as well. Many horse owners will be accustomed to using Rescue Remedy, which contains five

of Dr Bach's flower substances. These address five different mental states, any of which might arise as a consequence of trauma. These substances – for example, Rock-rose, Clematis, or Star of Bethlehem – can nevertheless be used individually to treat terror, or extreme fright (Rock-rose), indifference or absent-mindedness (Clematis), mental or physical shock (Star of Bethlehem). Like the list of homoeopathic remedies, Dr Bach's flower remedies, along with their pictures of mental symptoms, are contained in a *Materia Medica*.

Healing
In the treatment of back disorders, there is certainly a place for using the skills of a spiritual or hands-on healer. Healing is the ultimate form of energy medicine and it can be very effective. Horses are very responsive to healing and readily absorb the healing energy, especially when they have experienced long-term debilitating musculoskeletal problems. Relaxation of the body and mind are good tonics for any athlete, including the horse. No one can focus wholeheartedly on athletic performance if the mind is distracted by pain. Healing can be appropriate at any time, but it is particularly beneficial for horses with back disorders.

Alternative medicine, medicine that deals with the movement of energy, is often dismissed as quackery, and any therapeutic success is put down to the effects of auto-suggestion. However, not long ago, the smallest part of the universe was considered to be the atom; we now know that it isn't. Man has discovered particles far smaller than he ever imagined; and the possibilities of energy transference are completely overwhelming. This makes energy medicine the treatment of the future, not the past, even though others discovered its benefits thousands of years ago. Before dismissing this kind of medicine out of hand, it is worth considering just one small definition by one of the greatest scientists of our time:

'A virtual particle [is] a particle that can never be directly detected, but whose existence does have measurable effects.'
Professor Stephen Hawking, *A Brief History of Time*

6 Rehabilitation

Horses are not very efficient utilizers of grassland. Throughout evolution they have had to compete for a place on the plains with the more complex stomachs of ruminants. For this reason, horses browse for anything up to sixteen hours a day, and often cover distances of many miles. They continue to demonstrate this behaviour even in the confines of a small paddock where there is hardly a blade of grass to be seen. The horse therefore naturally spends a great deal of time with his body-weight over the forehand. The forelimbs of the horse are attached to the body wall only by connective tissue and muscle: this is sufficient to support the horse's body in the slow methodical rhythm of grazing. In flight, however, the horse has the ability

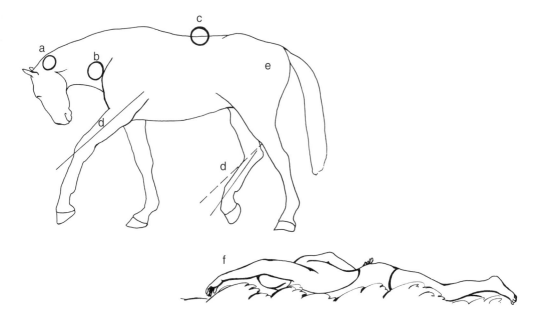

Horses learn to pull themselves along with the forelimbs, either through lack of education or because they have back problems. They become overdeveloped in the areas marked a and b, remain weak under the saddle at c, are unable to achieve the same angle of stride in the hind limbs as in the forelimbs d, and never develop the muscles of the hind quarters e. Their action resembles f, a swimmer doing the crawl.

to transfer his bodyweight onto the quarters, lightening the load on the forehand and protecting the forelimbs from concussion. Much of the horse's body language involves elevated paces, made possible by the extension and flexion of the spinal column, again protecting the forelimbs from the effects of overloading. In a natural situation, the horse moves within the specifications laid down by evolution. In addition to which, his muscles soften when he is eating, but their tone increases with the rush of adrenalin, when there is fear or excitement.

When the horse comes into a man-made environment, the demands on his musculoskeletal system change dramatically. He may be asked to cover the ground at speed, carrying the full weight of a rider almost directly over the shoulder-blades; or he may be asked to produce the kind of elevated paces with which he would intimidate another horse, yet do so in a totally relaxed and obedient way. In the wild, horses perform movements for a purpose, and these movements usually have a powerful emotional driving force. Yet a competition horse has to reproduce these movements without the support of this emotional drive. We are not asking the horse to carry out movements that are not part of his evolutionary repertoire. What we *are* doing is to impose conditions on these movements, and it is this that makes enormous demands on the horse's musculoskeletal system.

The horse's back is not only his drive shaft, it is part of his suspension. In general equine veterinary practice, a great deal of time is spent investigating lamenesses. Of these, a high percentage will be lamenesses affecting the forelimbs and, in particular, those arising from stress or concussion. Splints, sore shins, tendon and suspensory apparatus strain, ring bone, side bone, navicular syndrome, sesamoiditis, windgalls, pedal-bone fractures, stress fractures in the cannon bone – these are only a few of the diagnoses, and that is only going as far as the knee! It just goes to show how vulnerable the forelimbs of the horse are, and how basically ill-designed they are for the purpose of carrying a human being almost directly on top of them. That is, unless the horse really uses his back. Horses with all sorts of forelimb problems, from degenerative joint disease to legacies of old injuries, *can* be ridden, and often competitively, provided they are supple and soft through their backs. If the horse's back is kept constantly 'well-tuned', it is amazing how many problems in the front and hind limbs can be overcome, and just how much pain can be avoided.

An athletic career brings with it an inevitable accumulation of small stresses and strains, which together result in symptoms of gradual wear and tear. All horses are athletes, even if they only carry their humans round the lanes for an hour or so. To some this can be as demanding as a steeplechase. Then, there is the ageing process. Keeping the horse's back young may not be the secret of eternal youth, but it goes a long way towards reducing many other signs of ageing.

Rehabilitating the horse's back after illness, or just maintaining its suppleness as the horse gets older, involves a substantial amount of work from the ground, such as long-reining and lungeing. In addition, there is a variety of simple stretching exercises, which can be carried out in the stable before and after the horse has been exercised, and which help to relieve stiffness and tension in the horse's muscles. These can be used as a valuable form of 'occupational therapy' for horses that have to be box-rested after surgery. They ensure the horse's back doesn't stiffen and become uncomfortable as a result of standing in a confined space for most of the day.

Working a horse from the ground can be stimulating. It gives a different insight into the horse's movements, and leads to the establishment of a partnership based on mental rapport, rather than physical control. Nevertheless, rehabilitation work is demanding and time-consuming. In the time it takes to massage the horse thoroughly (that is, proper grooming, not a quick flick over with a brush!), run through the stretching exercises, tack the horse up with all the accoutrements for lungeing or long-reining, work effectively, perhaps with weights on a limb, possibly over poles on the ground, bring the horse back into the stable, undress him, groom him thoroughly (again), do some more stretches, give any medication, stand him under a heat lamp, carry out any other form of physiotherapy, rug him up, make his bed, check his feet . . . most people would simply have thrown a saddle on their horses and ridden them – probably several times over! However, a back that receives attention to detail is a back that will be capable of lasting athletic performance, and a back that will become strong, expressive and, at the same time, responsive to the rider.

The principles of rehabilitation are based on the three 'R's:

Revive
Restore
Re-educate

The process of reviving and restoring the back will have been initiated by the medical therapies. Whether it was the surgeon's knife, the acupuncturist's needles, or the healer's hands which got the ball rolling, the momentum of repair now has to be carried through into the phase of correcting the horse's movements. Once we are as sure as possible – through our own observations and the advice of the professionals – that the horse's back has reached the stage where it is *able* to carry out low-level gymnastic movements, it is time to address the dynamic problems that will have arisen as a consequence of the original disorder.

There is considerable variation in the way horses respond to back pain, or back problems. Horses with spinous process disorders may find it uncomfortable to rein back, they may flatten their backs over a jump, rush their fences generally, widen their stance in the hind limbs in certain movements, or develop changing degrees of unlevelness in any limb, depending on the type of work they are asked to do. There appear to be no absolute certainties when it comes to diagnosis. This is why the whole question of back pain, or problem, is so open to challenge by horse people from different equestrian disciplines. Everybody's expectations are different and, inevitably, so are their powers of perception. However, even though there are few movements that are absolutely diagnostic for back disorders, there are some that indicate that the back you see before you is a back in need of help:

At walk
• Reluctance to relax the neck, and stretch downwards.
• Swishing the tail or carrying the tail to one side.
• Holding the lower back stiffly, so that

the quarters appear to 'waddle'. (This may be more obvious on a downwards slope.)
• Difficulty in reining back.
• Dropping a hip, or occasionally collapsing with a forelimb.

At trot

Because of the diagonal nature of the stride sequence, and the characteristic moment of suspension between the diagonal strides, symptoms of back disorders are likely to be more obvious in trot than elsewhere.
• There is no clear two-beat rhythm: the horse appears to run along the ground, with little or no lift of the back.
• The horse finds it difficult, or impossible, to change his length bend, for example when going from one circle to another.
• Unlevelness when the rider changes his weight from one diagonal stride to the other.
• Widening of the hind limbs when the trot stride is lengthened.
• Going above the bit, and hollowing the mid-back.
• Repeated attempts to stretch the neck down, and run with the nose along the ground. This can be mistaken for the horse's ability to work 'long and low'. Horses should be allowed to relax their toplines at regular intervals in their schooling sessions: horses with back disorders tend to want to do this all the time.
• Inability to push off with the flat surface of the hind foot: the horse pushes himself forwards by toeing into the ground.
• The action of the hind limbs is passive, and the horse pulls himself along with the forelimbs: these horses are usually overdeveloped in their shoulders, but poorly muscled behind.

At canter

• Inability to canter on one particular lead.
• Constantly changing legs at canter, usually in favour of the same leading leg.
• Going disunited.
• Lack of forward 'jump', and hollow in the back.
• Consistently falling out of canter on one particular rein.
• Using the hind limbs together as though they were one single limb.
• Bolting.

In all the above examples, the back may not be the fundamental cause, but it will definitely be contributing to the overall locomotor disorder. It will need to be included in any rehabilitation programme before there can be a complete resolution to the problem.

Movement is generated by the nerve-cells in the brain and the spinal cord, in response to feedback from the muscles. The length of each muscle, its level of contraction and tone, are constantly measured against those of its opposing and supporting muscle groups. From the moment a foal gets on to its feet, each experiment in movement is stored and then gradually updated as the foal becomes more practised in organizing his limbs. This process never ceases, even when the foal eventually reaches maturity and his basic repertoire of movements is well established. All adult animals add to this repertoire, and this later becomes the basis for any form of athletic training. In a perfect world, all the nuances of movement that we add to our basic palette would be performed with the same degree of ease and elasticity.

Unfortunately, the slightest tensions or presence of low-grade injuries lead to modifications in the movements, which significantly change the overall balance of the body. These modifications are stored in the brain alongside the basic repertoire. Whenever the body is presented with a particular situation, they may be recalled as a first response. For example, a horse that has learnt to pull himself along on the forehand because of a badly fitting saddle, will respond in exactly the same way if the painful stimulus is reintroduced, even though he may have been working quite happily under a well-fitting saddle in the meantime. A horse that has developed a muscle spasm in the lumbar back to take the concussion away from a front foot with a painful abscess, will respond in the same way each time he experiences pain in that same foot, for whatever reason. Therefore, in rehabilitating backs, it is *not enough* just to restore the tissues to health and function; the whole back has to be re-educated, and the correct sequence of movements put in the place of the incorrect modifications. Remember, these incorrect responses will always be there; it is probably not possible actually to delete them, especially when the disorder has been long standing. But if the horse is retrained with absolute consistency, they can be more or less 'buried'. It becomes more and more difficult for the horse to recall them

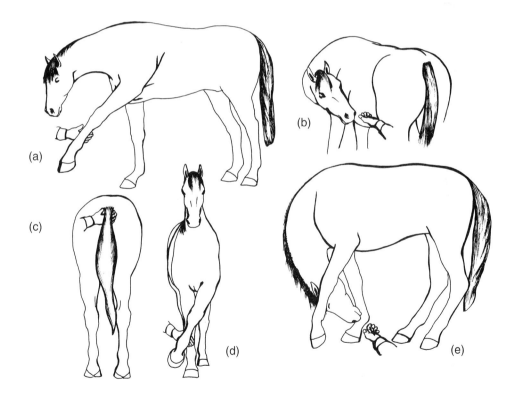

Stretching excercises. Passive stretching of a, the forelimb; b, the neck; c, the gluteal and lower muscles by pulling the tail; d, the forelimb across the mid-line; e, the lumbar portion of the back by offering a carrot from underneath the horse's chest.

101

because the correct way of going is continually put at the top of the brain's list!

A programme of rehabilitation and management will include the following:

- Stretching exercises.
- Remedial shoeing.
- Long-reining.
- Lungeing.
- Remedial saddle-fitting.
- Daily management (flooring, bedding, feeding techniques, grooming, rugs, turnout).
- Riding.

STRETCHING EXERCISES

The first step to ensuring that the horse does not perpetuate acquired incorrect movement patterns, in spite of the fact that he is capable of moving correctly, is to carry out a simple sequence of stretches on a daily basis. These exercises accustom the horse to relaxing parts of his back and limbs, which he might otherwise still try to guard, and counteract any tensions and stiffness that might creep in as he begins to resume regular exercise. Areas of the horse's body that are most likely to tighten up during the development of a back disorder (and therefore prone to tension when the horse first comes back into work) are:

- Either side of the poll.
- At the base of the neck.
- Across the withers.
- Behind the shoulder-blades.
- In the loins.

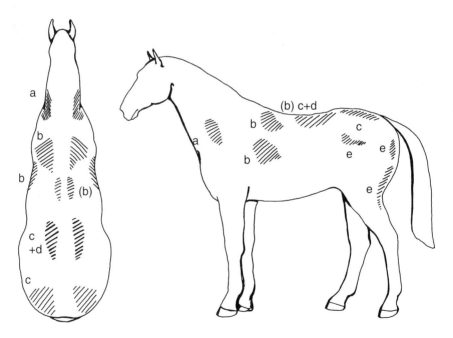

Areas of musculature affected by the different passive stretching excercises: a, neck stretches; b, forelimb stretches; c, tail pull; d, a carrot from between the forelegs; e, three-point dance with the hind limbs.

• In the quarters above the base of the tail.

In all cases the stretches should apply traction, but they should not be forceful. The intention is not to manipulate but simply to increase the range of mobility. Wait until the horse is relaxed and balanced before carrying out any movements. If the horse is attentive, he will make his own mental connection with the exercises, which will be useful during the later stages of schooling.

Forelimb Stretches

Exercise 1
Stand in front of the horse. Lift the forelimb and extend it towards you as though you were freeing the girth area after putting on the saddle. Wait until the horse has balanced himself over his quarters, then pull the limb towards you with a gentle but definite tug. Then let the horse replace the leg on the floor. Repeat two or three times. This exercise helps to stretch the muscles along the side of the horse's ribcage and behind the top of the shoulder-blades. A variation of the exercise is to pull the limb across the mid-line, which stretches the trapezius and latissimus dorsi muscles around the shoulder-blades.

Exercise 2
Pick up the forelimb as though you were going to pick out the feet. Gently rotate the foot two or three times clockwise, then anticlockwise. Repeat these small rotations for each joint: 1. pastern; 2. fetlock;

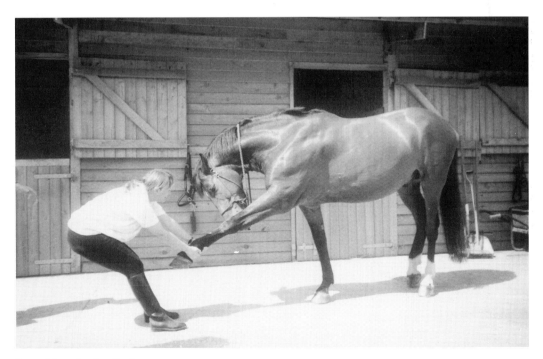

Stretching the forelimb.

3. knee (carpal joint); 4. elbow and shoulder combined. These rotations supple the joints, encourage the circulation, and help the production of joint fluid. They also have a relaxing effect on the pectoral muscles, which often become very tight in horses that go predominantly on the forehand.

Hindlimb Stretches

Rotations of the hind limb are carried out in the same way as for the forelimbs. Extending the hind-limb joints is also possible, but quite hard work! An effective variation is to carry out a three-point 'dance' with each hind leg.

Point 1
Stand alongside the horse, facing the tail, and pick up the hind foot, flexing the hind limb. Then bring the leg towards you, and place the toe on the ground as far forwards under the belly as the horse is able to reach. This stretches the muscles down the back of the leg.

Point 2
Pick up the foot again and direct the limb outwards, again placing the toe on the ground as far to the side as the horse finds comfortable. This stretches the muscles in the groin.

Point 3
Pick up the hind limb and extend it as far backwards as possible, until the horse can just touch the ground with his toe. This stretches the muscles down the front of the hind limb. Many horses find this the most difficult part, but if you use the verbal commands of the numbers, they accept the entire, three-part sequence more readily. This exercise can be carried

out two or three times at each session, with the object of increasing the degree of extension a little at a time.

Back and Neck Stretches

For some of these exercises, you will need either a carrot or a small wad of hay. The horse should fix whatever you offer him with his teeth, and this can be used to apply a small degree of traction to the body.

Exercise 1
To begin with, stand the horse alongside a wall, which will prevent him from swinging his whole body round. Stand at the horse's hip and offer him the carrot. As he takes it, give a short pull so that the base of the neck on the opposite side has to stretch a degree more than it is already doing. If there is a restriction anywhere in the neck, the exercise can be carried out with changes to the height of the carrot to increase the mobility and range of movement. Turn the horse round so that his opposite side is parallel with the wall. Repeat the exercise from this side of the horse. Most horses are used to being fed from the left side, so there may be 'learning' difficulties when the exercise is carried out from the right-hand side. It is sometimes easy to jump to the conclusion that the horse can't flex his neck this way, when in reality he just doesn't know that he can.

Exercise 2
Take another carrot. Stand at the horse's side, facing his head. Offer the carrot to the horse from a point on the ground underneath the mid-line of the chest, approximately where the girth would be.

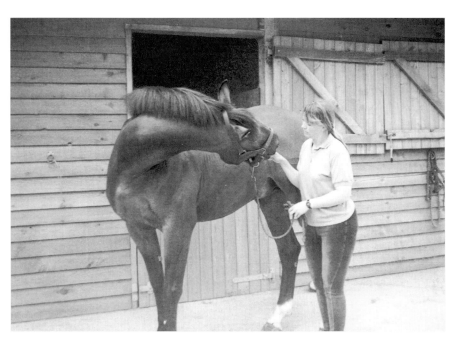

Stretching the base of the neck.

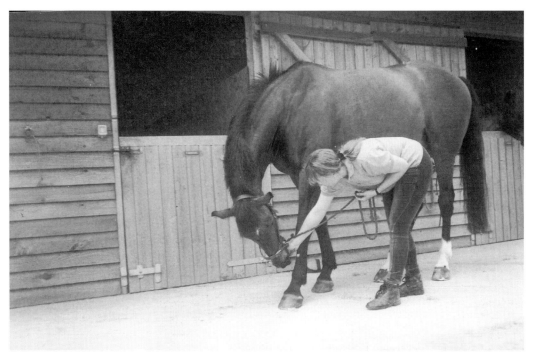

Introducing the 'carrot between the legs' exercise.

There again many horses at first think this is a lot of effort to go to in order to receive a titbit, and they need to be taught that their heads and necks really do go in this direction. Repeat the exercise while standing on the other side of the horse, in case he is inclined to cheat by dropping a foreleg. This is a wonderful exercise for stretching the whole topline, particularly the muscles of the loins and over the sacro-iliac junction.

Exercise 3
Finally, take the dock of the tail in both hands. Wait until the horse relaxes, then give the tail two or three short but firm pulls towards you. There should be a small ripple in the gluteal muscles of the quarters, that is, in the large muscle bulk between the point of the hip and the highest point of the spine (as seen from behind the horse).

A variation on this method is to place your fingers on the mid-point of both these muscles and pull your fingers down towards you, exerting a fair degree of pressure on the muscles as you go. The horse should first flex his hind limbs, then round his back all the way through the loins. Large or very well-muscled horses, sometimes do not respond to finger pressure alone; they may need the stimulus of blunt instruments to produce a response: use the ends of blunt spurs held in each hand, or the ends of two ball-point pens, for example.

These exercises can be done effectively

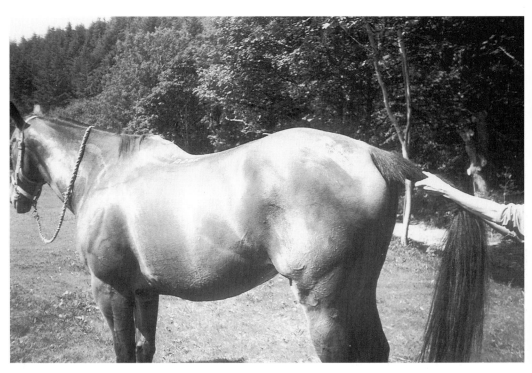

The tail pull.

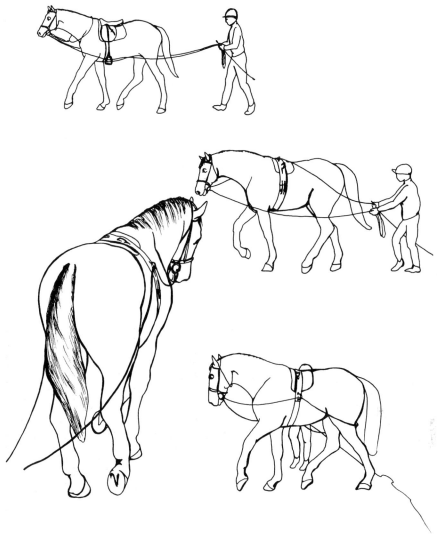

Different methods of long-reining.

and correctly in about five minutes. They should be used both before and after exercise. Even for horses with no apparent locomotor problems, a quick run through some or all of these stretches reduces the time necessary for warming up in schooling, and gives information as to any residual problems from training the day before.

LONG-REINING

There are a lot of misconceptions about long-reining: some people only associate it with training a young horse to be roadworthy; others think you have to be an associate of the Spanish Riding School to carry it out proficiently. There *are* in-between levels, and if you have learnt to

107

use the reins while sitting on the horse, you can certainly do the same thing, walking behind him.

There are two reasons for introducing a horse that has had a back disorder to exercise using long-reins:

1. The horse is taught to go forwards with confidence and self-carriage: these qualities are often lost when a horse experiences back problems or pain.

2. It gives the potential rider a good visual indication of how the horse moves through the whole length of his back: many riders will feel that a horse is moving awkwardly under saddle, without necessarily being able to interpret the movement's significance. Watching the horse walk away from you is a useful aid to diagnosis.

There is an additional psychological bonus to long-reining, which should not be underestimated. Many horses are long-reined before they are ridden. It's generally a time when the world is still in order and everything the horse is learning is new and exciting. Returning to this phase of the horse's basic education can help to rebuild his confidence and re-establish his trust, simply because (in most cases) he has no negative memories of this period in his life. Horses with back disorders can be very depressed because they are unable to express themselves as nature intended. The art of long-reining is not to be a back-seat driver, but to support the horse when he makes decisions and let him know that he can take on the world without self-doubt or insecurity.

There are a variety of styles of long-reining. In England it is traditional to loop the long-reins through the stirrups of the saddle, and walk several yards behind the horse. The contact on the bit is light, and the emphasis will be on encouraging the horse to go forwards fluently and boldly (round country lanes, or around a big field). Gradually, simple changes of rein can be introduced, using the touch of the long-reins against the horse's flanks to create a small degree of length bend. Depending on the original cause of the back disorder, it might not be appropriate to introduce the saddle, in which case a breaking roller might be more diplomatic. Choose one with low rings, or a good selection of rings at different heights for later lungeing, and pad well underneath. A breaking roller can exert just as much pressure across the withers as a saddle, and compresses the muscles around the shoulder-blades. If the horse is hollow behind the withers, pad these areas out as well, otherwise the whole exercise will be counter-productive. The additional support of loosely fitting side-reins may be a good insurance policy if you are long-reining alone along the roads. At this stage they should serve no other function.

Once the horse is moving freely within the long-rein frame, it is possible to be a bit more adventurous. (By this time the trainer will have become accustomed to holding several loops of line in each hand, will also know that the horse is not going to kick – actually very few do – and will have established a system of communication with basic commands, knowing what to expect from the horse in return.) By moving closer to the horse's quarters, either directly behind or a little to one side, it is possible to take up more weight from the contact to the horse's mouth. It is absolutely essential that the horse still goes forwards and does not begin to get 'stuck' in his movements, or worse still drop behind the bit.

Impulsion is more difficult to develop from the ground than in riding because you cannot reinforce the forwards movement with your seat and legs. In long-reining, it will be a combination of judicious use of the schooling whip, vocal commands and body language, that keeps the horse moving onto the bit. Smaller circles and lateral movements can be introduced, making sure the horse is balanced on the outside rein, and that there is softness on the inside rein. If necessary 'give away' the inside rein at short intervals to let the horse stretch through the base of the neck, whilst maintaining the contact and support on the outside rein.

It is quite likely that the horse will try to adopt incorrect ways of going, even on the long-reins, when asked to perform certain movements, such as going up or down hill, or making transitions. (These are his tried and trusted ways of getting himself out of trouble, or previously avoiding pain.) The trainer's hands must be sympathetic, but they must also be effective. Don't hesitate to increase the roundness of the topline for short interludes by asking for more collection, but remember to give the horse time to relax and stretch as well.

Incorrect movements include:

• Going above the bit and dipping the back. (This happens surprisingly little if the reins are carried at the correct height.)
• Lateral stiffness at the poll.
• Hollowing one side of the mid-back.
• Dropping a hip or jerking it upwards.
• Bringing one hind leg across the midline to avoid putting the whole weight on a (possibly) weaker limb.

'Kinks' tend to establish themselves along the topline when there is weakness. The more powerful side of the back takes over and dominates the production of power form the quarters, regardless of whether the other side of the back is 'sound' or not. Begin to counteract this response by introducing lateral movements, flexing the dominant side, and lengthening the weak side. When the 'strong' side has relaxed, change the direction of bend so that this side now has to stretch, and the weak side has to take the lead. As with lungeing and riding, be critical of your own posture while long-reining. Now is the time to practise relaxing your own shoulders and softening the elbow and wrist joints, without having to think about your seat and leg position in the saddle. Practise lengthening your own frame upwards through the spine to the top of your head, stretching your neck and walking lightly without collapsing either hip. If you have ridden the horse you are about to retrain, you have probably developed several kinks, too, to accommodate the horse's increasing lack of balance. Both horse and rider need to start with a clean sheet!

The length of time necessary for schooling from the ground will depend on the nature of the original disorder. As a general guideline, half an hour's work daily for three months will give you a back that is sufficiently well muscled and stabilized to go into dressage work at novice level. After one month of long-reining, the horse is probably ready to be hacked out, on a light contact, for one hour three times a week. After two months, the long-reining could possibly be replaced by lungeing, and interspersed with hacking, to give the horse variety.

A horse that has had a back disorder is a horse that has suffered a blow both to his physical framework and to his personality. Long-reining is about rekindling the horse's interest in his surroundings, helping him to find mental security, and generally bringing him back to life. Occasionally there may be misunderstandings: the horse and the reins will become dreadfully entangled, and you will suddenly have before you a trussed-up chicken! It doesn't matter: just quietly unravel the horse and start again. The horse is usually a bit surprised but afterwards pretty forgiving. If he continues to misbehave, or you feel he needs added interest, ask him to step over different configurations of poles. Use fan-shaped arrangements to change the length of stride, or raise the poles in alternate directions to encourage him to pick up his feet. This gently flexes all the joints through the limbs and is both suppling, relaxing and strengthening.

We should not expect the horse to do something under saddle that he is not capable of doing on his own. Therefore the more proficient he becomes in his gymnastic work without the rider, the more confident he is going to be once the rider is back in the saddle.

LUNGEING

How to lunge effectively is probably the most controversial question in general horsemanship. Do you lunge off a head-collar, a cavesson, or a bridle? Do you use side-reins, a chambon or any other balancing device? Do you work on big circles, little circles, or are continual circles generally bad for the horse anyway? Is lungeing a matter of whizzing the horse round on the end of a line, and trying to stop yourself going dizzy at the same time?

The horse benefits from lungeing only if you know what you are trying to achieve, and if you are working with equipment which you fully understand. If you can't see the effect you are producing then lungeing may not be for you. However, if you know what you are aiming for, this positive approach certainly transmits itself to the horse. Most horses seem to enjoy their lunge sessions, provided they are not carried out *ad nauseam*.

What can be achieved by lungeing:

* Rhythm and balance.
* Length bend.
* Confidence in accepting the bit.
* Transferal of weight to the quarters, and lightening the forehand.
* Stretching and strengthening of the back muscles.

Long-reining the horse can also develop these qualities, but for some people the degree of skill required to long-rein the horse successfully may seem too demanding. Long-reining certainly requires a greater amount of personal energy!

What is more difficult to achieve on the lunge:

* Control over the degree of length bend: some horses do not automatically change the bend of the quarters just because they have changed direction with the forehand, particularly if the mid-back is weak. Others forget to change the flexion of the poll when they change rein, which makes them appear lame.
* Adequate lift of the back: if the horse has been accustomed to flattening his back, especially in trot, he may not go forwards sufficiently on the lunge to really engage the hindquarters and arch the mid-back and loins.

Whatever the preferred method for lungeing, or the type of equipment used, there are two essential ingredients to success:

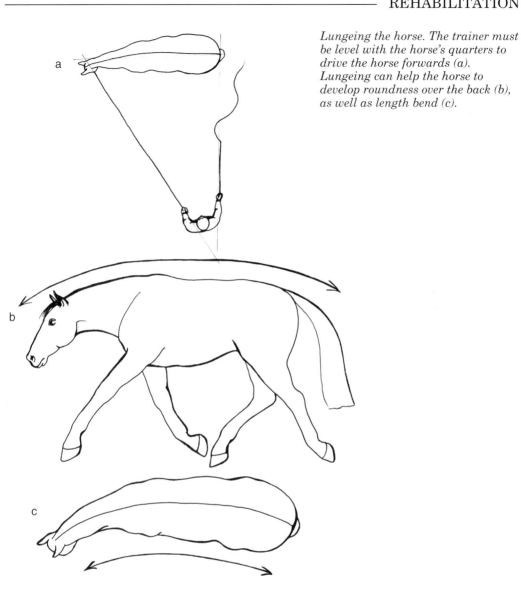

Lungeing the horse. The trainer must be level with the horse's quarters to drive the horse forwards (a). Lungeing can help the horse to develop roundness over the back (b), as well as length bend (c).

1. The horse *must* be driven from behind.
2. The hand holding the lunge line *must not* restrict the forward movement.

Therefore the commonest faults are:

• The whip hand is passive.
• The hand on the rein is tense, usually pulling downwards or outwards from the trainer's body.
• The trainer is positioned incorrectly to the horse's body – in front of the movement rather than with or behind.

To begin with, many horses fall into the circle or pull away from the trainer, which leads to all manner of gesticulations (flicking the whip at the horse's body, or flapping the lunge-line) in an effort to get the horse to describe a neat circle. Lungeing obeys the law of centrifugal force: if the horse is going forwards he will move outwards; if he slows down and is out of balance he will fall inwards. Horses need a warm-up period on the lunge, just as much as they do under saddle. Don't expect a perfect circle to begin with; wait until the horse has relaxed into a steady rhythm and is prepared to let you move level with the quarters. From this point the trainer can begin to drive the horse forwards with the whip, and the circle can become any size you want it to be.

Some trainers have criticized the use of lungeing as a training method because the horse is always on a bend, and this is thought to put additional strain on the joints. This does not have to be the case: once the horse is being driven forwards, and the contact on the bit is light but communicative, the horse can be directed along the length of the school, so that circles can be interspersed with straight lines.

Regardless of the specific lungeing equipment, your basic 'ground plan' in relation to the moving horse should be that of a right-angled triangle. The line from your body along the lunge-whip to the horse's quarters, and the line from the horse's hind feet to his forefeet, form the right angle. The lunge-line makes the third and sloping side of the triangle. How you carry the lunge-whip will depend on the horse's history; the lower and more quietly it can be used, the better, but it must be effective. The arm holding the lunge-line should be flexed and the hand carried, if possible, lightly in front of your body. A soft wrist is just as important here as it is in riding: a tight wrist is capable of inhibiting the forwards movement of a horse, even at twenty paces!

Choice of Equipment

Each item of lungeing equipment has its strengths and weaknesses. There is only one particular method of fixing the lunge-line that has distinct disadvantages for the horse, especially after a back disorder, and that is of passing the rein from the outside bit-ring, over the poll to the inside bit ring and then to the trainer's hand. Horses are sensitive to pressure at the poll.

This method is sometimes used to encourage the horse to lower his head carriage. However, the length bend of the horse's body on the lunge depends both on the position of the quarters and the poll. If the horse tightens at the poll because of unequal sidewards pressure, he may find it difficult to keep his balance through the length of his body, and build up many unwelcome tensions along the back as a result. Each piece of lungeing equipment must otherwise be taken on its own merits.

The Head

- Headcollar.
- Cavesson.
- Bridle.

The headcollar is suitable for the young horse, or one returning to work after a long convalescence. It imposes no restrictions, and allows the horse to experiment with his own self-carriage.

The cavesson can be a bit of a 'closed door' unless the horse is really asked to work from behind. He may be inhibited not only by the weight of the cavesson noseband, but by the optical effect of the lunge-rein being in front of his nose. However it is useful to begin with, in combination with side-reins on the bit-rings, to prevent the horse from getting conflicting messages to the bit should he temporarily lose his balance.

Lungeing off the bit-rings is controversial. Some people object to a possible nutcracker action of the bit on the bars of the horse's mouth. This can be avoided by using a double-jointed bit, such as a loose-ring French-link snaffle. This makes a good schooling bit for the horse under saddle as well. Passing the lunge-rein through the inside bit-ring and attaching it to the outside bit-ring, accustoms the horse to the increased contact on the outside rein, which he will need to develop in his ridden schooling, and it allows him to supple the inside line of his body without feeling restricted in his mouth.

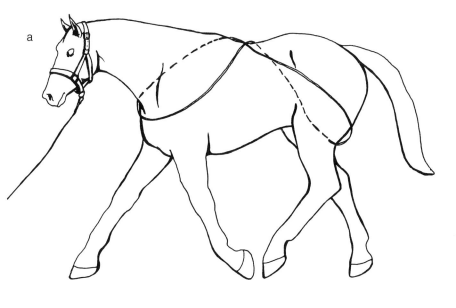

a

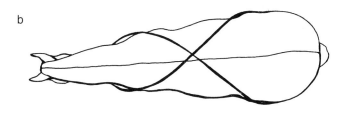

b

The figure-of-eight bandage; a modific-action of Linda Tellington-Jones' 'body rope'. a, side-view. b, viewed from above.

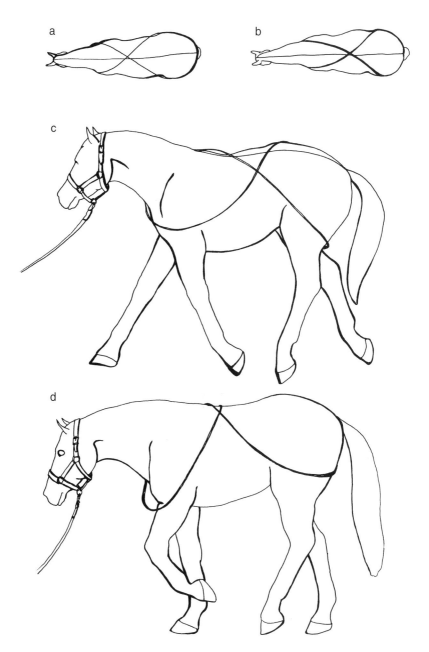

The figure-of-eight bandage applies gentle pressure to the hind limbs, encouraging the horse to step under, and bringing his back into contact with the cross-over point of the bandage. At the beginning, the cross-over point is just behind the withers, (a). As the horse shortens its frame the cross-over point should move further back, (b). This method also highlights peculiarities in the horse's movements, for example, dropping a hip, (c), or dropping the shoulders, (d).

114

Whichever system you prefer, as the horse develops self-carriage the weight of the lunge-line should begin to feel like a slender cotton thread in the trainer's hand.

The Body

- Surcingle or breaking roller.
- 'Body rope'.

The roller should have a good selection of rings at different heights, and be sufficiently stable. If there is too much movement, the horse will find it difficult to understand which movement of the side-reins, or similar, he should respond to. It should also be well padded at the withers and not exert undue pressure on the muscles around the shoulder-blades, as this will restrict the forelimb action. The roller is used for the attachment of side-reins, chambon strap or an additional lunge-line. The topmost rings (at the height of the withers) are used to imitate the position of the reins when held by the rider in the saddle. This needs very skilful handling and perhaps is best reserved for horses at an advanced level of schooling, rather than those recovering from back disorders.

The idea of the 'body rope' was developed in particular by Linda Tellington-Jones. A modification of it consists of two soft bandages, tied together and passed around the base of the neck, crossed over the horse's back, and looped around the hindquarters in a figure-of-eight configuration. The body rope provides an excellent way of making the horse aware of the connection between his hind limbs and his forehand. Many horses with back disorders learn to pull themselves along with the forelimbs, and are unaware of what the back and quarters are really doing. The horse moves away from the gentle touch of the rope around the hind legs, and in doing so begins to arch his back, bringing it into contact with the cross-over point of the rope. For horses that have had a great deal of pain in the mid-back, especially that associated with ill-fitting saddles, this is a useful means of mildly desensitizing the back without losing the lift and impulsion generated by the hind limbs. As the horse becomes more balanced and shortens his frame, the cross-over point of the rope automatically moves backwards away from the withers, which is a good indication of the horse's changing centre of gravity. When this happens, the length of body rope will need adjusting.

Balancing aids

- Side-reins.
- Chambon.
- Double lunge.

Horses with back disorders develop one or more of the following difficulties:

- They can't go forwards.
- They go forwards on the forehand.
- They lose the ability to lift and round their backs.
- They lose the sense of length bend.

Apart from the neck vertebrae, the spine does not have as much flexibility as we might think when compared to the considerable changes in posture that can be achieved by the muscles. Therefore, the ability to work through and over the back, to generate elevation and impulsion, are all down to muscular training, without which the horse will find it very difficult to sustain his balance under the rider.

Horses move in a certain way either because they have been taught to do so, or because they have never been taught to do otherwise. With a little support and (sometimes quite a lot of) patience, most horses will experiment with their way of going until it becomes apparent to them that this new way is acceptable to their human partner. This is a great asset when it comes to retraining or rebuilding the back muscles. Whilst there are advantages to lungeing a horse off a headcollar with no restrictions, it is often necessary to give the horse a suggestion as to what you are actually after, and this means introducing a balancing aid. However, it

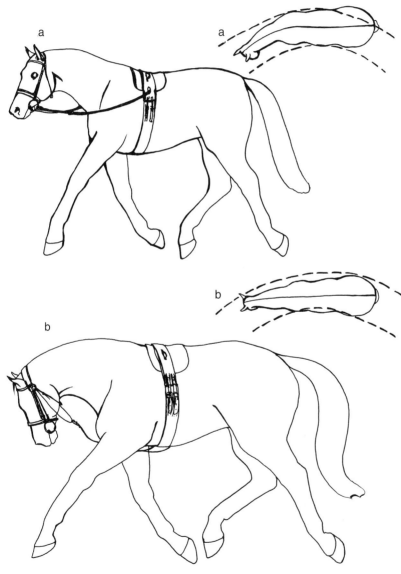

Side-reins create length bend only as far as the shoulders (a). A chambon gives the horse no help whatsoever with length bend, but is excellent for developing the top line.

116

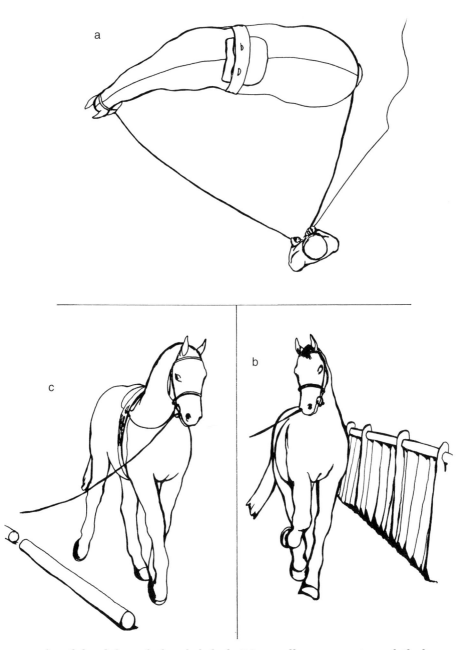

To encourage length bend through the whole body it is usually necessary to work the horse on a double lunge, (a). Horses lean inwards when the optical framework is on the outside of the lungeing circle, (b). This can be corrected by lungeing the horse around the outside of a pole circle on the ground. The horse stays more upright and the weight is more evenly distributed between the inner and outer limbs.

117

must be underlined, that no balancing aids are effective unless the horse is really driven forwards from behind; otherwise, they become just another burden to be avoided – and evaded!

Side-reins can be used to introduce a light contact on the bit, to increase the degree of contact as the horse becomes more balanced and, when used at different lengths, to create a sense of neck bend which is supported by the outside rein, just as it would be in riding. If a horse has been uncomfortable in his back, he will almost certainly have built up some form of resistance to the bit because he won't have been able to soften his whole body in response to its presence. The tension may be in the jaw, at the poll, at the base of the neck in the shoulder, or even somewhere down a hind leg, but it will have to be over-come if the horse is to make a full recovery.

The only disadvantage to side-reins is that the length bend is not necessarily carried through the whole body. To achieve this with some horses it is neces-sary to use a second lunge-line which passes around the horse's quarters. This second lunge is excellent for increasing the engagement of the hind legs by applying a little pressure, while giving the outside frame of the horse sufficient support on the circle. Work on a double lunge then becomes a logical extension of the work introduced using the 'body rope'.

The chambon comprises a headpiece, and a continuous line which passes from one bit-ring through both rings of the head-piece, to the bit-ring on the other side. This line forms a loop under the throat, which is linked to a single strap attached between the forelegs to the surcingle. When the horse raises his head, the bit is lifted in the mouth; when he lowers the head again, the bit returns to its comfortable position.

At first glance, it appears that the chambon places pressure on the poll, and so causes the horse to run on the forehand. However, the headpiece is fixed, so in fact the action is on the mouth, and the horse actually lightens his forehand in response to his own impulsion. The greatest effect is achieved when the chambon is used in conjunction with lengthened shoes on the hind feet. The horse pushes off with the entire bearing surface of the shoe, and the action is followed through, right the way up the hind limbs, along the back, under the shoulder-blades, to the base of the neck. Using the chambon, even on a once-weekly basis, is one of the most successful methods of strengthening the back muscles and of encouraging the horse to work over his back. The disadvantage is that it gives the horse no help at all with length bend.

Poles
The horse's balance can be improved not only by gymnastic training over poles on the ground, or over cavaletti, but also by the use of visual stimuli. Horses are normally lunged inside an arena or lungeing circle, where the optical barrier is on the outside. The horse leans, even if only marginally, away from the outer wall, so that on a circle the outer and inner limbs are loaded differently. Once the horse is carrying the rider's weight, leaning in on the corners, or on small circles, places an abnormal load on the inside legs, particularly the foreleg. This causes a shortened forelimb stride with soreness in the shoulder muscles. The horse can be trained, on the lunge, to keep an upright posture even on a circle; this is done by working him on the outside of a pole circle. An arrangement of poles on the ground, placed end to end to form a ring,

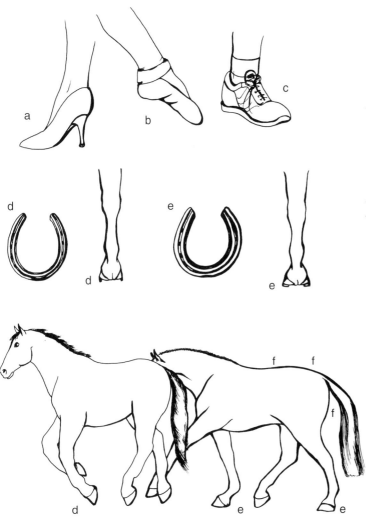

All shoes have an affect on balance. Humans would expect to use the shoes a, b, and c, for different purposes. A narrow horse-shoe (d) gives the horse's limbs little support, compared to a broad-based shoe (e). A horse will use a narrow shoe to cut into the ground for better grip, but this does not mean that he will also use his back (d).

The horse can use the broader-based shoe to push himself off the ground with every stride (e) and this automatically engages his back and quarters (f).

is sufficient to encourage the horse to load the inside and outside lengths of his body equally, rather than trying to be a motorbike! Alternating circles from outside to inside the pole ring is a good way of combining a suppling exercise with a balancing one. In combination with the chambon, this kind of visual support helps the horse to achieve length bend as well as lift. A fan-shaped arrangement of trotting poles, raised on alternate sides adds variety to the lunge work, and increases the gymnastic potential of all the other techniques.

REMEDIAL SHOEING

Unless you have access to plenty of favourable off-road going (and not just a sand school), there will come a time in the rehabilitation programme when the horse will have to be shod. The ultimate choice of shoe will depend on what the horse is going to do when he is back in full ridden work. In the meantime, the shoes are going to be as much a part of the overall prescription as any of the other healing therapies. In fact the foot balance and shoeing are the cornerstones of all the training to come, once the back is fully functional.

The horse's foot is a piece of precision engineering. The way in which the horn tubules grow down from the coronary band depends on the movement pattern of the entire limb. Any restrictions – wherever they are – that change the fluency of movement through the limb, alter the direction of growth of the horn tubules, and ultimately change the shape of the foot.

The most severe examples of such a development are seen in the collapsed heels of a flat-footed horse, or the contracted heels of a horse with boxy feet. However, there are more subtle restrictions which change the side-to-side balance of the foot, and which gradually stress the lateral or medial hoof walls. Such changes often have their origins in muscular restrictions along the horse's topline, which prevent the hoof from breaking over at the optimum moment. The horn growth cannot respond correctly to what are actually very narrow loading specifications, and the shape of the hoof becomes distorted.

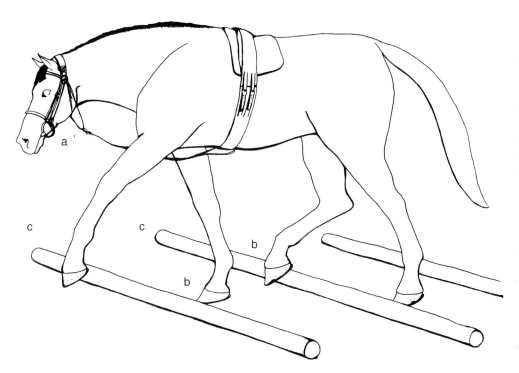

To develop suppleness, and strength in the horse's back, try a combination of chambon (a), broad webbed shoes (b), and work over trotting poles (c).

A horse that has experienced a back disorder needs a wide bearing surface under his feet. If he is asked to balance himself on very narrow rims of metal too soon into the rehabilitation programme, he will simply tighten up again and renew all the responses that led to the problem in the first place. This becomes even more important if the horse is going to do a significant amount of work on an artificial schooling surface. A narrow fullered shoe is designed for cutting into the ground while hunting, not for keeping your balance at canter half-pass, or even on a series of (20m) circles at working trot in a sand school. The horse constantly has to save himself from falling over the edge of this type of shoe, which puts an unbelievable amount of stress on the joints of the pastern and fetlock, and eventually tightens the withers and the entire back.

However accurate the old adage 'no foot, no horse', it is almost certainly as true to say 'no back, no foot'. For this reason, broad webbed shoes with good, and long, heel support are the basic requirements for rehabilitation exercises, both on the front feet and the back feet. The reason for using a broad webbed shoe on the hind feet, is that many horses resort to hooking their hind toes into the ground to propel themselves forwards. On a schooling surface the horse appears to be 'tracking up', but he is not really pushing off with the surface of the hind foot, only with his toe. The engagement of the hind limbs in this way is not sufficient to create a good lift of the back, right through to the shoulders. These horses are adequately – though not powerfully – muscled in the quarters, and they are generally hollow behind the withers.

Provided you are absolutely certain the horse can respond with his back,

increasing the bearing surface and the length of the shoes on the hind feet will gradually improve the musculature of the whole topline, even whilst the horse is walking round the field. A word of caution, though: many farriers are reluctant to shoe long because of the increased risk of the horse's pulling off a shoe. Horses recovering from back disorders are likely to be unbalanced and, yes, they will pull off a shoe until they are established on their 'new feet'. Promise your farrier faithfully to use overreach boots, and the farrier will generally be more receptive to adding half an inch of length to the shoe.

It takes about three weeks for any remedial shoeing to attain its optimum effect. It very much depends on how quickly the horse is prepared to experiment with his own body. Some horses are quick to adapt, and are willing to explore different movement possibilities. Other horses are incredibly obstinate, and particularly unwilling to let the shoes exert their full effect. After the optimum time the foot growth will start to unbalance the shoes, and the horse may not be able to work quite as successfully. It will be up to the farrier to assess whether he can develop the shoeing towards encouraging even more response from the horse's muscles, or whether the horse is sufficiently established. In some cases, it might take as long as twelve weeks before the horse is able to cope with a more demanding shoe.

As a general principle, the level of training of the horse's topline should be held in place by the shoeing, and changes in the shoeing should allow for renewed development of the horse's topline. This reciprocal function becomes most apparent when the horse begins the ridden stage of his remedial work.

121

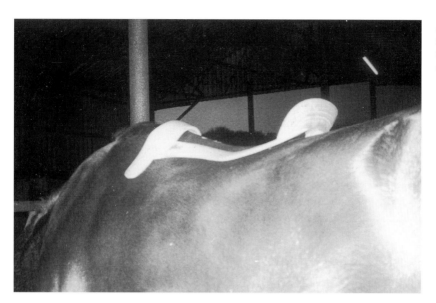

Even today the saddle is still an upholstered seat on a fixed frame.

THE SADDLE

The basic concept of the saddle has not changed for thousands of years. It remains to this day an upholstered seat on a fixed frame, which is strapped around the horse's chest and which provides some point of anchorage for the rider's feet. Yet in spite of having fulfilled these specifications for centuries, the saddle still remains the greatest experiment in the history of horsemanship. Even in the last ten years, emphasis on different elements of the saddle's shape has changed, and although the weight distribution of saddle and rider can now be diagnosed by computer, the search for the perfect solution is by no means over.

The problem lies in the fact that the horse's back needs to move, but the rider's body needs security. Furthermore, the shape of the horse's back and the rider's seat are similar, but not that similar. Therefore the purpose of the saddle is to bring the two shapes together, allowing

the horse to move to his best advantage, and the rider to remain in close contact in order to give precise commands. In short, the saddle must be an interface. There is now a consensus as to the general requirements of a well-fitting saddle, but opinions still differ considerably as to the details. Perhaps it may one day be possible to construct a saddle using some high-tech viscous material that adapts one surface to the horse's body, while moulding its other surface to the rider's seat, without the need for a fixed frame to retain its shape. Until such time, however, a saddle has to meet the following anatomical and locomotor needs of the horse:

• The saddle should not press or rest on the spinous processes anywhere along the thoracic spine.
• It should give reasonable clearance of the withers, both in height *and* width.
• The arch of the tree must be wide enough to allow the shoulder-blades to

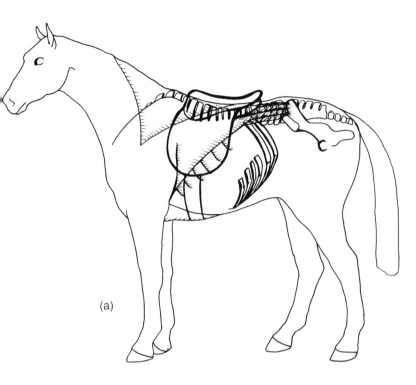

(a)

a) The saddle rests on a combination of bones and muscles.
b) The saddle also encloses vital organs in the chest.

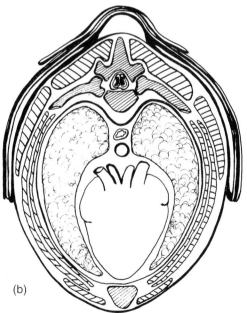

(b)

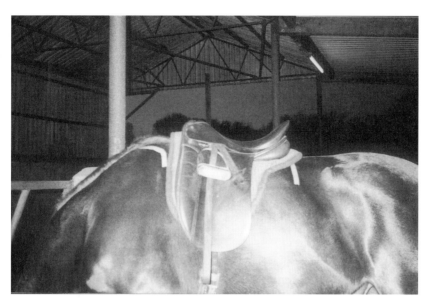

The saddle should not place the rider over the unsupported spine, nor interfere with the movement of the shoulder-blades.

rotate and the muscles over the shoulders to expand when the horse is working.
• The *entire* bearing surface should be in contact with the back muscles of the horse, distributing the rider's weight as evenly as possible.
• The consistency of the flocking in the weight-bearing panels should allow the back muscles to respond to the rider's aids through their *whole* length.
• The length of the saddle should not place the rider over the unsupported lumbar spine.
• The depth of the seat should not bring the rider's weight too close to the horse's shoulders.
• The girth attachments should keep the saddle balanced, but not restrict the movement of the shoulders.
• The buckles of the girth straps should not exert excessive pressure on the rib-cage, restricting the horse's breathing.
• The position of the stirrup-bars should not cause the saddle to pivot onto the horse's shoulders when the rider stands in the stirrups (when adopting a forward seat for jumping or fast work).

There are anatomical and locomotor considerations for the rider, too:

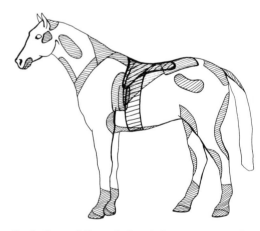

Both the saddle and the girth can cause pain by exerting uneven or excessive pressure. Yet there are many other areas which can become tense and eventually painful when the horse has to work in an ill-fitting saddle.

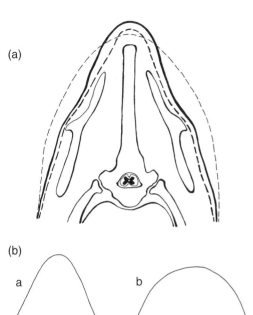

(a)

(b)

a   b

(a) A cross-section through the horse's withers, showing the possible variations in width.
(b) The arch of the saddle-tree should correspond to the width of the horse's withers. It should also match the withers' profile: a, more V-shaped, or b, more U-shaped.

• The seat of the saddle must accommodate the *whole* seat of the rider, both lengthways and sideways. This means taking into account the width of the rider's pelvis and its degree of rotation.
• The saddle should allow the rider to sit in the correct position for the particular equestrian discipline, and for the level of training.
• The stirrup-bars should allow the rider's leg to rest in the stirrups so that the lower leg is in line with the rider's body (in any discipline).
• The length of the side-panels should suit the length of the rider's leg and take into consideration the position of a long riding boot.

If there are not quite so many stringent requirements for the seat of the saddle as there are for its bearing surface, this is probably because it's the horse that is expected to move while being sat on, not the other way round!

A well-fitting saddle should meet the following minimum standards:

• The arch of the tree should match the width and slope of the horse's wither profile. There are two basic shapes of arch: one is shaped like an inverted V, the other like an inverted U. A narrowly built Thoroughbred may have V-shaped withers, while a cob may have U-shaped withers; the former may have long sloping shoulders, the latter short chunky ones. (Remember, this is only an example: there are obviously broad-shouldered Thoroughbreds as well as narrow-shouldered cobs.) Most

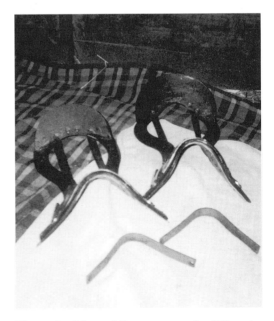

The arch of the saddle-tree comes in different width fittings, and different profiles.

125

V-shaped arches are inclined to have slight indentations between the top of the arch and the points of the tree. These tend to interfere with the movement of the shoulder-blade in any shape of horse. For this reason the U-shaped arch is to be preferred.

• The width fitting of the saddle should accommodate the horse as he *should* be when correctly muscled. Where there is muscle wastage around the withers, some form of substitute padding may be required to fill in the hollows until the horse has built up his profile through remedial exercises.

• The saddle should make best use of the back muscles available to provide a generous bearing surface. Gussets give the saddle stability either side of the spine.

• The flocking should be smooth, without lumps, bumps or hollows. Traditional flocking can be hard and lumpy, but otherwise holds its shape well. Pure wool flocking is very comfortable for the horse but compacts more quickly than the traditional flock. It needs regular checking and, if necessary, regular adjustment.

• The central channel should be wide enough to accommodate the dorsal spinous processes through the length of the whole saddle: the horse's spine does *not* get narrower towards the loins!

There is absolutely no doubt that the cause of very many back disorders is the fit of the saddle. In most cases, the problem begins as a response to uneven pressure. This causes loss of blood supply to the muscles and thus damage to the mechanical receptors underneath the skin, which leads to paralysis through compression of the motor nerves and, ultimately, to pain. In fact, once the pain receptors in the back have been activated, it is sometimes very difficult to switch them off again. Balance and weight distribution of the saddle are therefore of paramount importance.

Uneven and eventually harmful

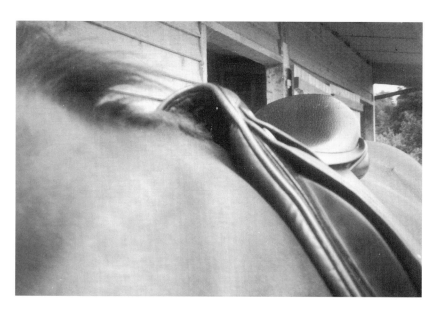

The arch of the tree must accommodate the width of the shoulders.

pressure to the horse's back can be caused by:

• The arch of the saddle, or thick seams of leather under the arch, rubbing on the top of the withers.
• The profile of the arch catching on the side of the withers as the horse bends his neck.
• Compression of the dorsal spinous processes by the weight-bearing panels (usually caused by overflocking).
• Compression of the dorsal spinous processes by the saddle moving across the spine.
• Asymmetry in the weight-bearing panels.
• Broken saddle-tree.
• Twisted saddle-tree.
• An exposed tree, when the central channel is too wide and the rider's weight forces the panels apart.
• Girth straps attached to the points of the tree, if this interferes with the rotation of the shoulder-blades.

• Areas, however small, of uneven flocking: either too much or too little.
• Stirrup-bars that are angled inwards towards the horse's back muscles.
• Girth buckles.

It is sometimes hard to imagine that an animal as big as a horse – and apparently of such robust stature – could find an area of increased pressure the size of an English pound coin so intolerable that he would change his whole way of going to avoid it, even rearing or napping. Yet, like the fairy story in which the princess could feel the presence of a pea through a pile of mattresses, the horse's back is extraordinarily sensitive. To the horse, anything that clamps onto your back and causes pain is a predator, and you either run away from it, fight it, or die!

There are now a multitude of back-saving devices on the market, which are designed to help the horse cope with the effects of saddle pressure. Many make use of new, synthetic, shock-absorbing materials

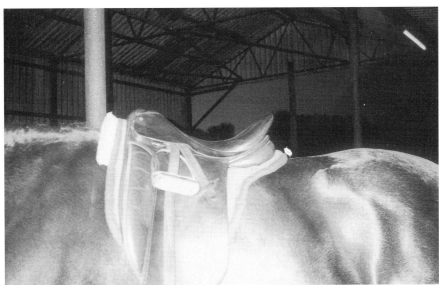

When there is muscle wastage the saddle must first be supported by other means – for example, a padded numnah and / or shoulder wedges.

(a) (b) (c)

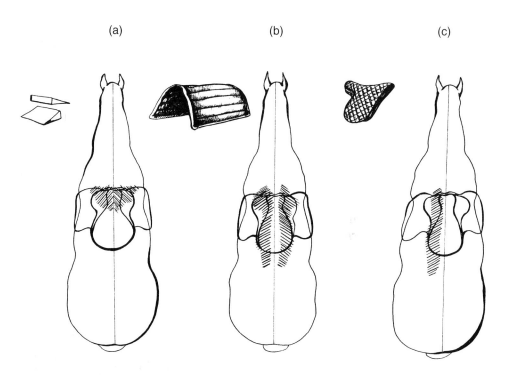

Muscles that have wasted through a previously incorrectly fitted saddle, must be recreated artificially to allow the horse to build up those muscles again. (a) For muscle loss under the points of the saddle-tree, use wedges made out of high-density foam. (b) For muscle loss under the saddle as a whole, use a thick, or even double-thick, numnah. (c) For muscle loss on one side of the back only, use a numnah doubled over.

(thank goodness that the American space programme spends so much time researching them!). However, the fact remains that a well-fitting saddle should be like well-fitting shoes. The more socks you try to stuff into badly fitting shoes in order to cushion the feet, the tighter and more uncomfortable they become. If the saddle fits correctly a thin cotton numnah should be all that's necessary. However, there are some occasions when the saddle may need extra support or cushioning, even if only on a temporary basis:

• If the horse has lost a great deal of muscle along the topline, the saddle should still be fitted to his intended shape, but the lacking muscle recreated by using one, or even several, thick numnahs.

• If the horse has muscle wastage along one side of his spine, do not be tempted to build up one side of the saddle – this just causes additional pressure, which is counter-productive. Instead, double over one numnah and place it under the saddle on the side where there is less muscle. The saddle will be in balance, and the horse can build up underneath.

• When the muscle wastage affects only the area immediately around the withers

– a very typical situation – make two wedges using high-density foam (any other type compresses too easily) and slip them under the arch of the saddle. These give the points of the tree something to rest on, without digging into the trapezius muscles, and they help to stop the saddle slipping forwards and bumping into the edge of the shoulder-blades. (Note that high-density foam can be irritant, so the wedges need a cotton cover.)

In most cases, the object of any rehabilitation programme is to return the horse's back to its full function. The rider needs to communicate with the horse through his seat, and should always be able to feel how the horse's back responds. However, in very arthritic horses that are realistically never going to regain any suppleness in the back, but that are quite happy to go out for gentle exercise, it is advisable to use a good, shock-absorbing material underneath the saddle, such as a gel pad or similar. The same is true for horses that round their backs excessively over a jump, so that the spine touches the tree of the saddle. Here, some form of protection becomes a necessity.

Disregarding the conventions of style and fashion, there is much to be said for the use of a Western saddle, especially in horses that are beginning to show signs of arthritis in the forelimbs. The same criteria of width and balance apply to the fitting of Western saddles as they do to

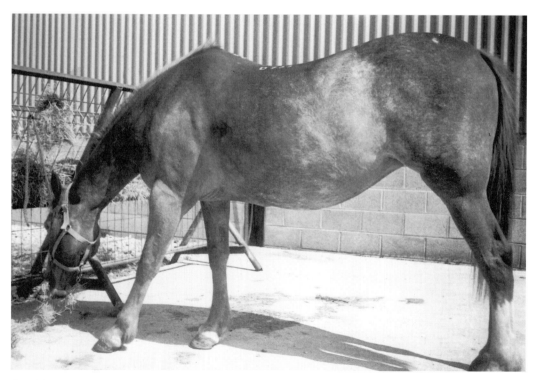

An older horse with a long and less well-supported back.

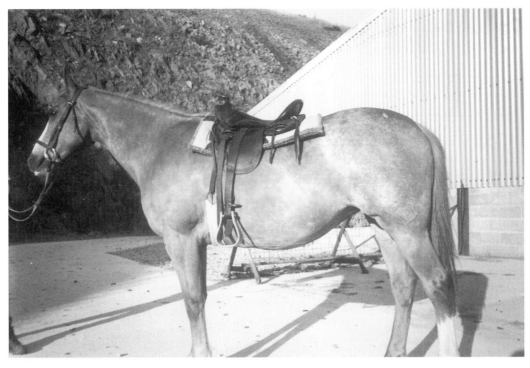

A possible saddle solution for the older arthritic horse: the Western saddle keeps the rider well away from the horse's forelimbs.

English ones. However, the advantage of the Western saddle is that it places the rider in the middle of the horse, keeping the rider's weight away from the forehand. It allows the rider's leg to rest in a natural position close to the intercostal nerves, which activate the belly muscles and allow the horse to step under with his hind legs. The contact between the rider's seat and the horse is surprising, considering the thickness of the saddle, and horses that otherwise stumbled and shuffled are able to move far more freely under a Western saddle because the rider is automatically in balance.

It is possible to have English saddles converted to a system whereby two independently moving panels are attached to the underside of the saddle, giving it an appearance similar to that of the Western saddle. The choice of materials for these panels, as well as their final design, is still experimental, but there are certainly horses that have been cured of lameness problems and back disorders simply by using this type of saddle conversion.

7 Daily Management

If you got out of bed every morning feeling as though you had spent the whole night lying on some medieval instrument of torture, you would probably at least consider buying a new bed. The horse deserves the same consideration, especially if he has suffered from a back disorder. The conventional life-style of the horse – alternating between an enclosed stable and a small acreage of grazing – is about as far removed from his natural state as it would be for us if we were asked to hang upside down all day like a bat in a cave. We might load horses on to aeroplanes, transport them half-way round the world, and then expect them to win prestigious prizes, but the fact remains that short bursts of exercise, however intensive, followed by long periods of standing on the spot, is not what the horse was originally designed to do. In his natural environment, the horse is on the move for much of the day (and night). Long periods of eating alternate with relatively short periods of rest. (If you have ever spent a night in a stable yard, you will have had first-hand experience of this behaviour pattern.) Movement may be only slow and unadventurous, but it still means that the engine of the horse's musculoskeletal system is always gently ticking over; it is never completely 'cold'

should the horse suddenly need to exert himself in flight.

STABLING

Few people can provide their horses with an environment that allows them constant freedom of movement all the year round. Probably an open barn system comes closest, and horses kept in such a system are generally at ease physically and (particularly) mentally. However, space is usually at a premium, and it therefore falls to the horse person to ensure that the horse's musculoskeletal system is properly prepared before any strenuous exercise is attempted. This doesn't just mean an adequate warm-up time during ridden work. It actually embraces the whole system of management, from the way the horse stands in the stable to eat his hay, to the type of feed he is on, who his neighbours are, what sort of rugs he wears, and how long he spends in the field.

The design of the stable, and the position of the feed bowl, manger or haynet have considerable influence on the horse's well-being. Horses are not cave dwellers; in the wild they would naturally be able to change their grazing or sleeping positions according to the positions of other horses

131

in their social groups. In a stable yard, it is quite possible for a horse to feel intimidated by a more dominant neighbour, yet have to eat his hay in this neighbour's close proximity. This situation leads to a mental conflict between the necessity to eat, and the instinct to eat somewhere else! The horse expresses this anxiety by holding himself tightly along the back, and he does not necessarily relax even when he leaves the stable to be ridden.

In addition there are two features of a typical stable that contribute in particular to the (dis)comfort of the horse. One is the slope of the stable floor; the other is the height of his forage. If the horse has to stand for several hours with his quarters higher than his withers, for example, because the stable floor slopes down towards his hay, he will be continually compressing the dorsal spinous processes in the mid-back. These will eventually become sore, if not seriously inflamed. This discomfort is certainly increased if

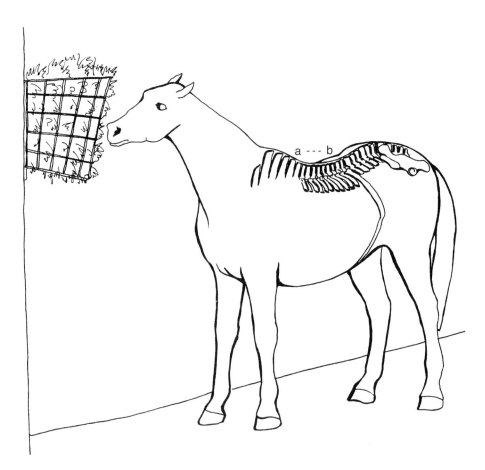

A horse that stands for long hours with a hollow back, is in danger of compressing the dorsal spinous processes in the mid-back, a . . . b.

the horse has to eat hay from any fixture, such as a haynet or rack, that is raised above the height of his shoulders. It may be hygienic and practical to feed forage in this way, but it isn't physiologically sound.

Young horses are especially vulnerable if fed from high racks. They have a tendency to grow higher at the croup before they catch up at the withers, and therefore may be standing for long hours with hollow backs, particularly during winter stabling. Problems in their backs are often not discovered until they are broken in, which may not be until the skeleton is fully developed.

Haynets are not usually hung high enough to cause the horse's back direct damage, but they are often placed so that the horse has to twist his neck to reach his hay. A horse may have to repeat the same one-sided rotational movement of his neck many times over before he has finished his hay ration for one day. There are possibilities here for quite bizarre muscle development, which affects the horse's balance under saddle. For the comfort of the back (as well as to reduce the inhalation of dust and spores) feed forage from a clean floor, or from a container placed at ground level. 'Landscape' the floor of the stable, for example by using deep litter, to relieve pressure on the horse's mid-back whilst he is eating.

FEEDING

There are several ways in which the choice of feed itself influences the horse's back. Firstly, there is general body condition. The spinal nerves are embedded in the long back muscles. If those muscles are poorly developed or wasted, the nerve-fibres will lie only just under the skin's surface and will be vulnerable to pressure. It can take months to rebuild muscle, even with daily training. It is sometimes better to encourage the build-up of an insulating layer of fat by generous feeding, rather than risk damage to the nerve-endings. As the exercise load increases the fat is gradually replaced by muscle. The overall shape of the back doesn't change, which is an advantage when wanting to fit a saddle right at the beginning of a rehabilitation programme: the horse's shape is already defined even though it may be replaced by one of more athletic substance later on.

Performance horses constantly tread a thin line between maintaining peak energy levels and going into metabolic 'melt down', otherwise known as azoturia. Through the study of applied kinesiology, it is now known that individual feed substances can also have an effect on muscles to the point of significantly reducing their mechanical strength, even though they don't cause complete instability of the muscle membrane as in azoturia. For example, sugars with different molecular structures, as well as certain trace elements, can have just such an effect. The result is a weakening of key elements in the locomotor system, which very often disturbs the balance of the back. Diagnosis by kinesiology is not yet widely used in horses, but given the variety of ingredients which find their way into horse rations, it may well prove to be a valuable tool in the investigation of some locomotor disorders.

It cannot be emphasized strongly enough that the relaxed suppleness of the horse's back depends a great deal on his mental state, and this is influenced by the basic components of his diet: proteins, carbohydrates, fats. Some proteins and carbohydrates are broken down by

133

digestive enzymes very quickly, and these give the horse immediate access to a large amount of energy. Some carbohydrates and fats release their energy much more slowly, so that it is available to the horse over a longer period of time. A horse that gets all his energy in a quick buzz is going to react differently from a horse on a slow energy release type of diet. Under the stress of competition a horse needs to draw on quick-release energy, whereas at other times this may simply make him fidgety and less compliant. The benefits of daily gymnastic training may be lost on a back which is continually wound up like a coiled spring, simply because it is being fuelled by a high-performance feed.

Feed stuffs that release energy slowly are likely to keep the horse warm over longer periods between feeds. Horses lose a lot of body heat through their backs, and there are many different shapes of back that need special consideration when it comes to keeping the back muscles warm and supple. Horses at the peak of fitness carry very little insulating fat, and they can quickly go from their optimum lean weight to being under weight if their backs get cold. In Thoroughbreds, with their high exposed withers and slender loins, it is difficult to keep weight on their toplines, because they feel the cold, more than we perhaps imagine. Horses with long backs, especially if they are a little hollow with age, can chill very easily when it rains heavily, because the water simply collects in the hollows. This is made worse if the horse has a thick winter coat: far from being a protection, the coat holds the moisture causing the horse to hollow even more as his back gets colder. A warm rug, or simply a water- and wind-proof New Zealand, helps to keep condition on the back and cuts down the cost of extra feeding.

GROOMING AND CLIPPING

It has become usual to clip horses as soon as autumn approaches, in order to reduce the amount of sweating during strenuous exercise, and to save time in grooming a thick coat caked in mud. There are even people who have such a strong dislike of mud that they never allow their horses to get down and have a good roll. Rolling is important, especially to horses that may be stabled for long periods. It helps to release small areas of tension which may have built up during exercise, and which are much less likely to dissipate if the horse is just standing still. (If a horse gets down and rolls immediately the saddle is removed, this is probably an indication that the saddle is causing discomfort.) Rolling enables the horse to manipulate his own spine, and correct small degrees of misalignment along the vertebrae. The way in which he rolls is often quite specific to the type of work the horse is doing, and it should be watched very carefully. It may be symptomatic of pleasure – or pain.

Although clipping and rugging is undoubtedly a convenience, a thorough groom is nevertheless an important part of the preparation for exercise. It stimulates the blood circulation in the capillary bed beneath the skin, massages the superficial muscles, and gives the handler vital information about the horse's readiness for the work to come. If the horse has lain awkwardly in his box, or slipped coming in from the field the day before, he may be locked in the neck or quarters, or have a twinge somewhere along his back. These things need attention *before* the horse is worked, rather than afterwards. There are many instances of horses being made to go through one day's strenuous exercise with minor ligament or muscle strain, only to be off work for many months afterwards with serious damage to their backs as a result.

Horses are inclined to be more demonstrative about areas of pain during grooming than they are under saddle where they can be more easily dominated. An obedient horse will struggle to perform to the best of his ability even with an injury: it is up to the human partner to interpret the horse's body language as early as possible in the dialogue of training, rather than let misunderstandings develop into a full-blown row. Thorough grooming *before and after* exercise is a way of opening up the conversation that is about to take place between trainer and horse, and then closing it again: a sort of 'Hello, how are you today?', followed by a 'Thank you for listening to me, and see you tomorrow'!

8 Riding

A book about the horse's back is inevitably a book about riding, since riding is the culmination of all our efforts on behalf of the horse's back in the first place. Driving horses can get back disorders – of that there can be no doubt – but they are generally allowed more gymnastic freedom than riding horses and can modify their way of going in the face of injury without having to support the weight of a rider. In fact, there are many horses that have to retire from ridden work because of irreparable damage to their backs, but apparently thoroughly enjoy a second career being driven.

Putting a collar around the horse's neck enabled prehistoric man to cultivate the soil more efficiently and to transport his goods further afield. Putting a saddle on the horse's back enabled the rider to wield more powerful weapons than he was able to do riding bareback, and to travel greater distances in the pursuit of more land. The prowess of an army and the skill of horse-riding became closely linked, and the art of horsemanship played no small part in the ventures of many conquering heroes throughout history. Today equestrian sports are all in some way derived from activities that were once intended to develop the skills of the military horseman and his horse. Athleticism, precision, and obedience are the cornerstones of competition now, just as they were once the keystone of military training, with one small difference: there is no longer any battle to be fought. The skills are taught entirely for their own sakes, and this significantly moves the goal-posts. The yardstick by which a horse's sporting achievement is measured now has no end. There are no ultimate conclusions to training: there are only the limitations of the horse's musculoskeletal system. Speed, height, degree of collection, and sustainability of collection make demands on the horse's frame like never before, and a crucial part of that frame depends on the strength and agility of the thoracolumbar spine.

Horses come in many shapes and sizes, and although many breeders are striving to produce the ideal conformation for a modern sports horse, one glance around any field of competitors will reveal that, thankfully, a great deal of variation is still possible. Evolution is a slow process, and when the demands for speed and elevation have reached their utmost, the only challenge left is precision. Again the ability to control and unfold power at split-second intervals stretches the horse's frame to the limits, a frame which, after all, takes its commands from the nerves of the spinal cord. Showjumping, eventing, dressage, even racing, are all nowadays precision sports; the moment of peak fitness has to be precise virtually to a day, the accuracy of movement timed to a degree.

Preparation of the horse for top-level competition has become extraordinarily scientific, combining the monitoring of blood gases with information gathered from exercise on treadmills, and gait analysis using force-plates in the ground. In fact, it is quite surprising that competition horses are not all required to carry on-board telemetry units, like racing cars. There is nothing wrong with making the best possible use of scientific data to improve the horse's performance, but at the end of the day it is a horse and not a machine we are dealing with. A top-class horse may have all the perfection of a highly tuned machine, but that does not mean it is no longer a living creature, a being of flesh and blood – and feelings.

Nearly everybody drives a car. We may not understand everything that goes on under the bonnet, but we all have a sense of power when we switch on the engine. This power is a reasonably obedient servant: it trundles when we want it to trundle, it can be exhilarating when we want to be exhilarated. In fact, the car is now such a sophisticated machine that it is capable of reflecting many idiosyncrasies in the human personality. However, there is no doubt that our living in a society dominated by the motor car

(a)

(b)

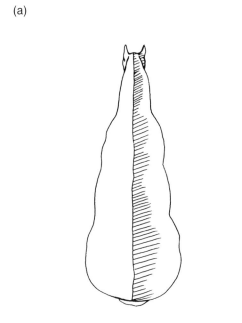
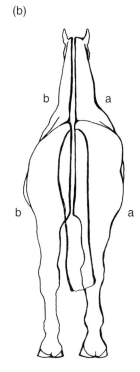

(a) Whether due to injury, or to the horse's personality, one side of the back can become dominant. (b) One side of the horse can be well-muscled and powerful (a,a), whilst the other side remains weak and lacks stability (b,b).

has changed our perception of the horse, and our awareness of the horse's movements. For example, saddlers are often asked to adjust saddles that slip to the left or right. More often than not, it is not the saddle that is out of balance, it is the horse; but it doesn't occur to the rider to examine this possibility through the medium of the saddle because he is far more used to sitting in the seat of a car, which is an inanimate machine. Yet if you *ask* that rider whether he has the same contact with the horse's back under both seatbones, he will be able to tell you that there is more contact on one side, less on the other. Ask the rider to become conscious of the movement of the horse's hip as it comes towards the seat bone on the weaker side, and he will find that the two sides of the back under the saddle begin to give equal support, and his hips move in unison with those of the horse. From the moment we sit in the saddle, it is important to remember that we are not just in charge of another vehicle, we are in charge of another body.

The ultimate thrill of riding is to feel that every moving part of the horse's body is an extension of your own: your legs are part of his hind legs, your hips part of his hips and back, your arms part of his forehand. The whole is controlled by two minds working in unison. So if, after riding, your back aches or your hips feel lop-sided, you can bet your life his do too! If one stirrup feels longer than the other, is it you or is it the horse? Does your horse need a chiropractor – or do you? There are a great many riders who know they are skeletally unlevel, who have perhaps one leg shorter than the other or an injury that prevents them from keeping both legs in a similar position. Yet they ride with equal-length stirrups, putting 60 per cent of their weight on one side of the horse's back and only 40 per cent on the other. For the horse that is a difference of 20 per cent, and *his* left and right bends are supposed to be the same!

The biggest dilemma for the rider at the end of this high-tech twentieth century is: do we *know* what we expect to feel when we sit astride the horse? The prevalence of back problems suggests that we don't: the search for their cure suggests that we'd like to.

Postscript

A book on the horse's back can have no ending: there is always another horse, just around the corner, with a back that has a problem as individual as the horse himself. One may draw on all the experience of treating similar cases, and still this next horse will require a nuance of treatment that one had not previously considered. It is a never-ending story of discovery.

There are many ways of understanding the horse's back, as a rider or trainer, as a therapist or a physician. The horse's back is like a musical instrument. It can be played in tune or out of tune, with feeling or without. When it gets damaged, it can be fixed quickly with a temporary repair job, or it can be painstakingly restored, like a valuable violin. There are many gifted 'restorers' of horses' backs, and my book would not have been possible without my having had the privilege of watching them work. This book is a summary of observations, made on behalf of the many friends who have helped me with the treatment of horses' backs: the McTimoney chiropractors, the physiotherapists, the healers, and some very special veterinary surgeons. If this book has helped in any way towards our understanding of the horse's back, perhaps it will also have helped towards our understanding of the horse.

Index